MAHOGANY

STEPS TO CUTTING, COLOURING AND FINISHING HAIR

Martin Gannon
and Richard Thompson

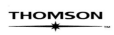

WELLA

MAHOGANY

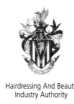
Hairdressing And Beauty
Industry Authority

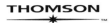

Mahogany - Steps to cutting, colouring and finishing hair

Copyright © Martin Gannon and Richard Thompson, 1997

The Thomson logo is a registered trademark used herein under license.

For more information, contact Thomson Learning, 50-51 Bedford Row,
London, WC1R 4LR or visit us on the World Wide Web at:
http://www.thomsonlearning.co.uk

British Library Cataloguing-in-Publication Data
A catalogue record for this book is available from the British Library

ISBN 1-86152-693-8

First published 1997 by Macmillan Press Ltd
Reprinted 2001 by Thomson Learning
Reprinted 2002 by Thomson

Printed by ZRINSKI d.d., Croatia

NOTE ABOUT PRONOUNS

Using 'he' or 'she' and 'him' or 'her' throughout the text would become cumbersome in a book such as this. For simplicity and ease of reading, therefore, we have generally used 'she' and 'her' except in passages concerned specifically with men's hairdressing.

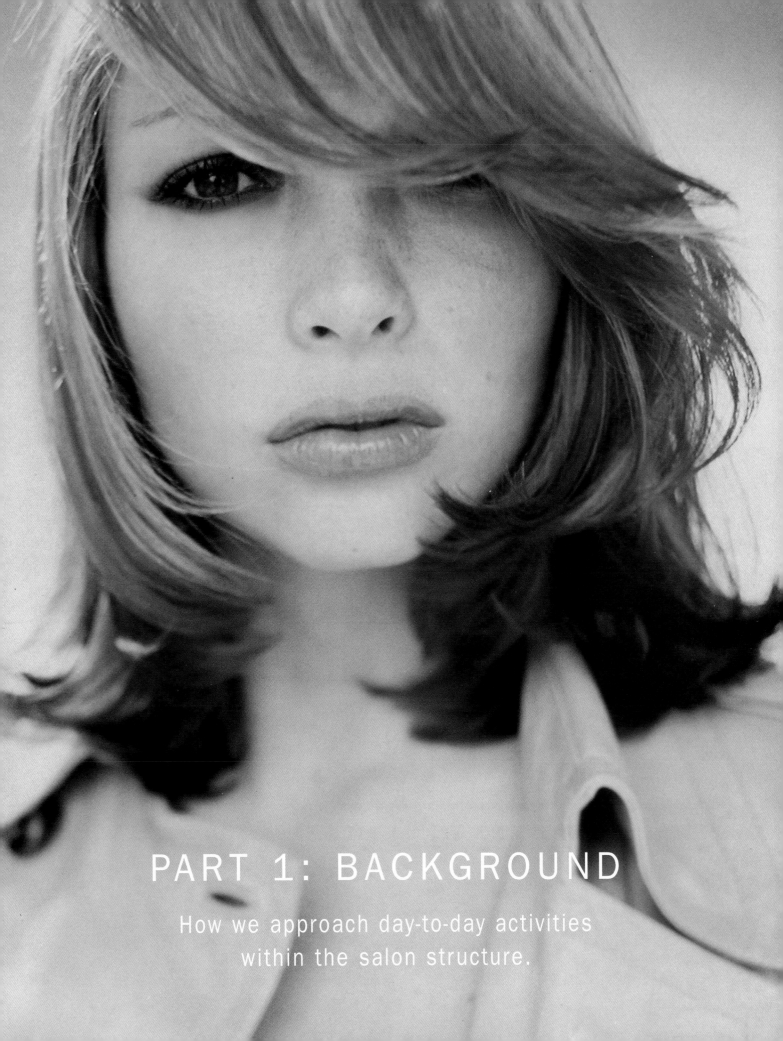

PART 1: BACKGROUND

How we approach day-to-day activities
within the salon structure.

SALON AMBIENCE

The ambience of a salon should be energetic and at the same time relaxing for the client. In order to create the right environment for both staff and clients, the following points should be considered.

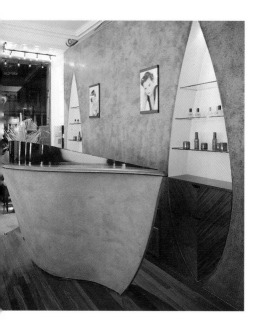

RECEPTION

The moment a client walks through your door she senses the ambience of the salon – the efficiency, the welcome, the images of the people working there, all these impressions are soon noted and subconsciously stored.

The reception may include a retail area offering a wide range of professional hair care products which will support and maintain clients' hair between salon visits. It should be attractive and uncluttered.

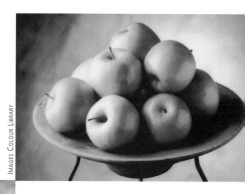

IMAGES COLOUR LIBRARY

IMAGES COLOUR LIBRARY

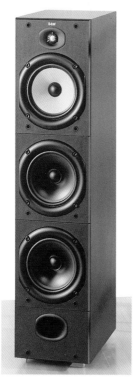

B & O LOUDSPEAKERS LTD

DECOR

The decoration of a salon is a matter of the owner's personal taste. However, the overall success of the salon's appearance will also be determined by an awareness of the clientele you want to attract, of what is acceptable to a variety of people and of what is fashionable in interior design.

MUSIC

Music is also very personal, but in a hairdressing salon where communication between stylist and client is of paramount importance, music should be interesting without being dominant. What type of music would suit your clientele? Will the music you choose help to create a relaxing or a stimulating environment?

Keep the speakers away from reception and position them high up so that no one has to sit in a direct blast of sound.

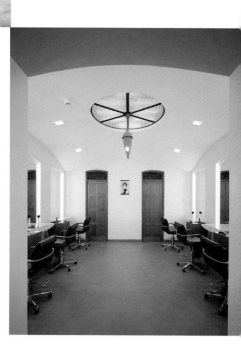

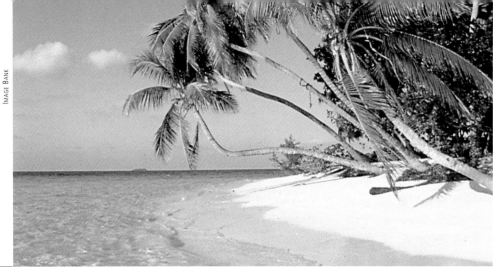

AIR CONDITIONING

Air conditioning removes negative ions, keeping the air fresh and
clean and free from unpleasant chemical odour and cigarette smoke
(if you allow smoking in the salon). It will also cool or heat the space.

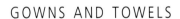

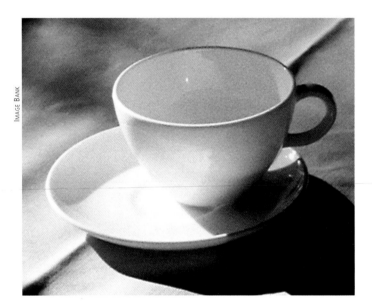

GOWNS AND TOWELS

Gowns should feel very comfortable, be
protective and fit all shapes and sizes. The best
are made of a silky drip-dry fabric. You should be
able to have the neck of a gown tight or loose
to facilitate cutting different lengths of hair.
Towels should be thickish and soft and large
enough to form a turban on the head – an
attractive and secure option to finish and present
a client in preparation for styling, colouring or
perming, and a more glamorous image for the
client. The comfort factor creates an attitude,
the attitude creates an overall ambience.

REFRESHMENTS

Teas, coffees, mineral water, juice – which should you offer? We find that
increasingly people are asking for herbal tea, decaffeinated coffee and
tea. We believe it is best to provide a varied but concise selection, served
in cups that are easy to stack, easy to carry and easy to hold.

PHILOSOPHY

WHAT IS THE MAHOGANY PHILOSOPHY AND WHY DO WE HAVE ONE?

It's probably more of a formula – the procedures we follow, everything we can possibly do to keep a loyal clientele.

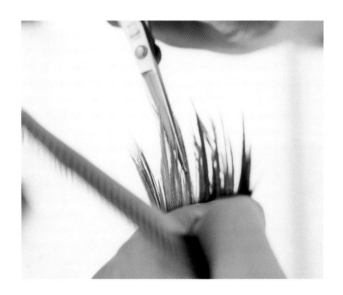

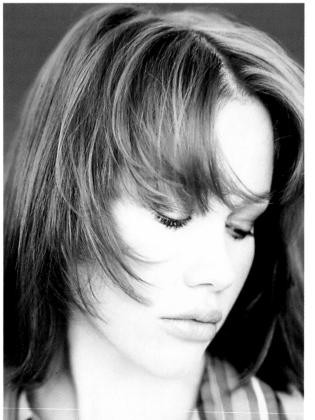

CUTTING

All Mahogany staff are trained within a system which consists of three-month modules over a two-year period. Each module covers a different aspect. Consistency of quality and procedure creates a confident, loyal clientele.

Let's take an example. Stylist Tom always cuts Miss Smith's hair, but Tom is away and Susie cuts it instead. Because all Mahogany stylists use just one pair of scissors to create a look and because they have all been trained within the same system, Miss Smith's hair will be cut using the same tools, and the same procedure. The client will feel that there is a consistency in procedure and technique and is more likely to be a happy client.

Now let's take another example. All the stylists in the salon use different tools for cutting hair – Tom uses scissors and a razor, Susie uses scissors and thinning scissors. Tom is away and Miss Smith, Tom's loyal client, goes to Susie. Instead of using a razor, Suzie uses thinning scissors. Immediately the client will feel unsure and will more than likely question this procedure. This will take away the confidence of both the client and the stylist. When Tom returns to work he is likely to have lost the client, or the client will complain to him about how the cut wasn't the same.

It is Mahogany's theory that under these circumstances a business cannot grow, because the client comes to depend on an individual stylist's experience not on the experience of the whole salon.

COLOUR

Hair colour is divided into depth and tone. Depth, also called base colour, indicates how light or dark the hair is, e.g. blonde or brown. Tone is the visual reflective quality of the colour, e.g. red or gold or ash.

In natural hair, two types of pigment are present: ashen pigments and warm pigments. The elongated molecules of ashen pigments appear as black or brown and are the easiest to remove when lightening the hair. The warm pigments are red and yellow. These molecules are more difficult to remove as they are smaller and spherical and are fused better into the hair structure.

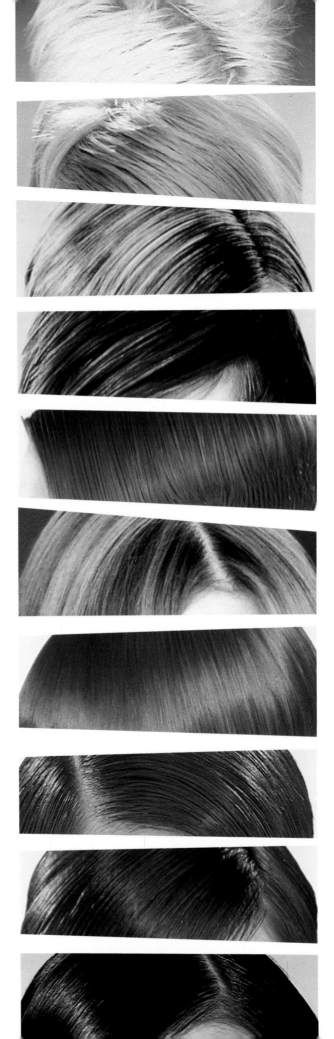

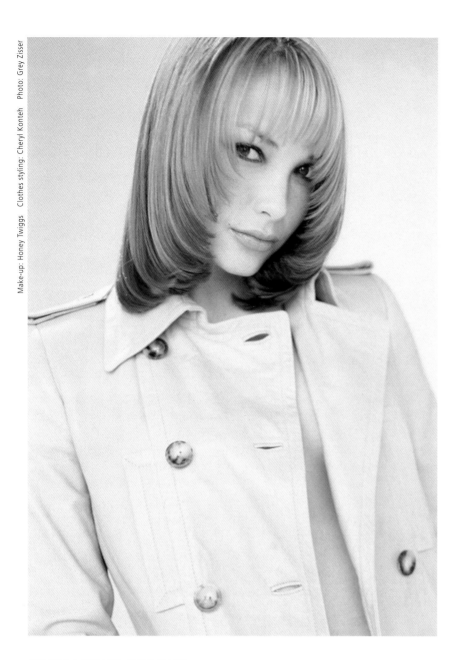

Make-up: Honey Twiggs   Clothes styling: Cheryl Konteh   Photo: Grey Zisser

PERMANENT COLOUR

Permanent colours, also known as para dyes, work by mimicking natural pigments and in some cases by masking them. They work by chemical reaction between the dye substance and hydrogen peroxide.

The dye contains the colouring agent and ammonia, also such additions as conditioning polymers, in an emulsion base. The ammonia has two functions. Firstly, it opens up the cuticle of the hair shaft to allow the colouring agent to enter the hair. Secondly, it activates the hydrogen peroxide, as hydrogen peroxide will only give up its oxygen in an alkaline state.

Once in the hair shaft, the free oxygen molecules join the colourless colouring molecules and they swell and the colour develops. Once swollen they become insoluble in water and too large to rinse from a normal hair shaft.

TEMPORARY COLOURS

These types of colour come in many forms. Most are applied to wet hair and they coat the hair's surface. The colour pigments are positively charged and are attracted to the negatively charged hair. The pigments are very often vegetable-based.

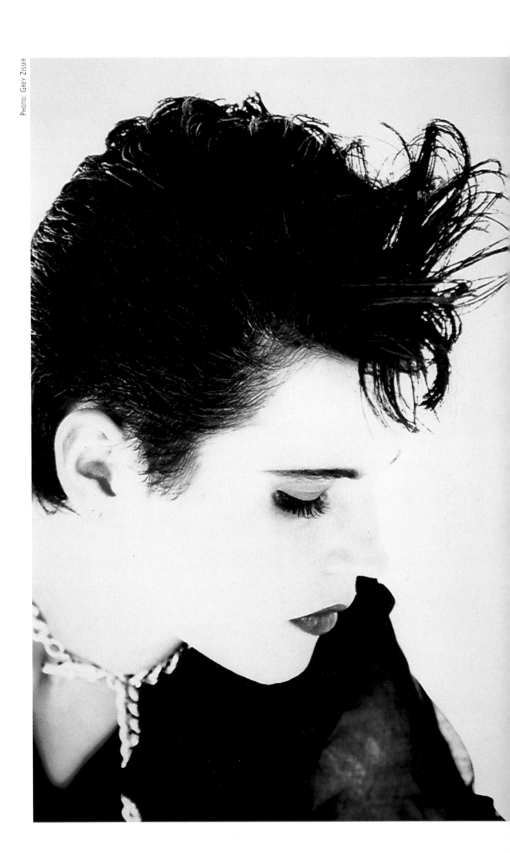

TIPS

• Temporary colours cannot change the base colour of the hair and will wash out of normal hair in 1 to 6 shampoos. They can be used to top up fading permanent colour between tints.

• Colour may be applied to the hair straight from an applicator bottle, but a tint bowl and brush is the preferred method because it looks more professional.

BLEACHING PRODUCTS

Bleach is basically an alkalising agent which, when added to hydrogen peroxide, releases the oxygen in the peroxide into the hair shaft. This breaks down the hair's natural pigmentation.

It comes in two basic forms – a powder or an oil emulsion. Powder bleach is the stronger of the two and is used widely for off-scalp processes such as highlighting. Adjusting the peroxide strength will alter the lifting ability of the bleach.

Oil emulsion works in the same way but it is a gentler lightening agent used for on-scalp application. The strength is adjusted by the addition of boosters.

Bleaches contain ammonia, ammonium hydroxide, ammonium persulfate silicates and sodium.

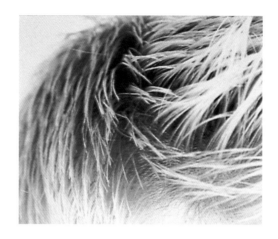

TIPS

● When you are bleaching regrowth, never re-apply bleach to other areas of the hair – there should be no overlap. Bleaching is a very strong chemical process and must be carried out with great care.

● Even a strong bleach may not remove all the yellow pigment and a toner may be used to cover this yellow.

● If you lift bleach to white it will not hold a toner.

TIPS

● Remember that the name tone on tone indicates that these colours add pigment to the hair and therefore you must be careful when choosing the right colour. Less than 50% grey, you should use a lighter base colour than the client's. For example, if the client's base colour is light brown, do not apply light brown – the result would be dark brown, as you have added pigment to the hair.

● It is common practice at Mahogany to colour a client's hair before the cut if the cut isn't going to be a total change, i.e. from long to short.

TONE ON TONE COLOURS

Tone on tone colours have largely replaced the older type of semi-permanent colours, which are now known as temporary colours. This is because of the modern habit of shampooing every day, which removes the old colour too quickly.

Unlike the older semis, tone on tone semis enter into the hair shaft to a greater degree, and produce stronger and longer-lasting colours.

They are mixed with a colour developer which contains hydrogen peroxide at between 2% and 4% and are applied to wet hair following a shampoo with a detoxifying cleanser.

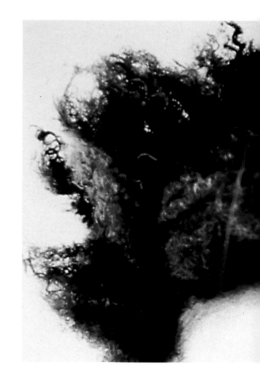

PART 2: TECHNIQUES

The basics to start from.

ONE LENGTH BOB

Precision-cut outline without graduation.

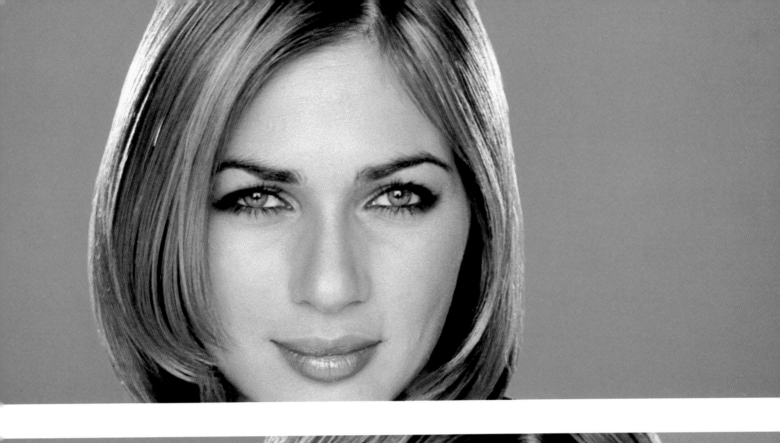
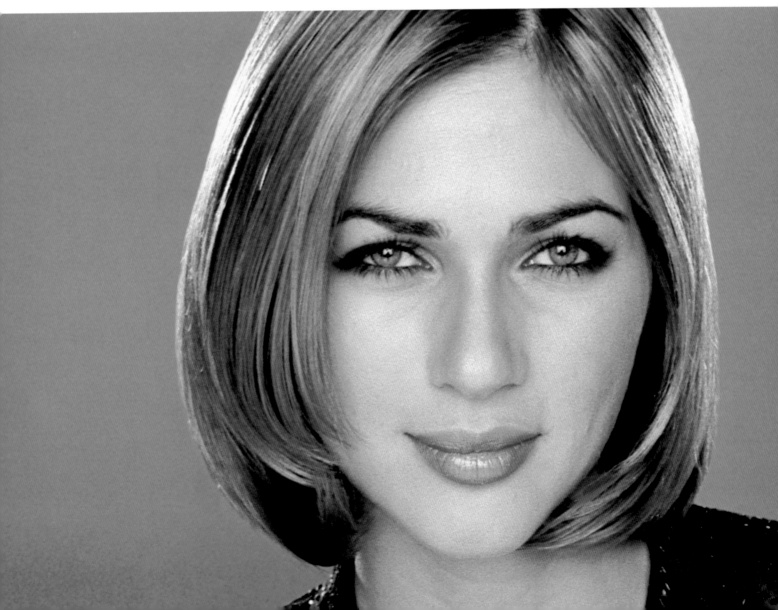

GRADUATED BOB (1)

Precision-cut outline with square graduation.

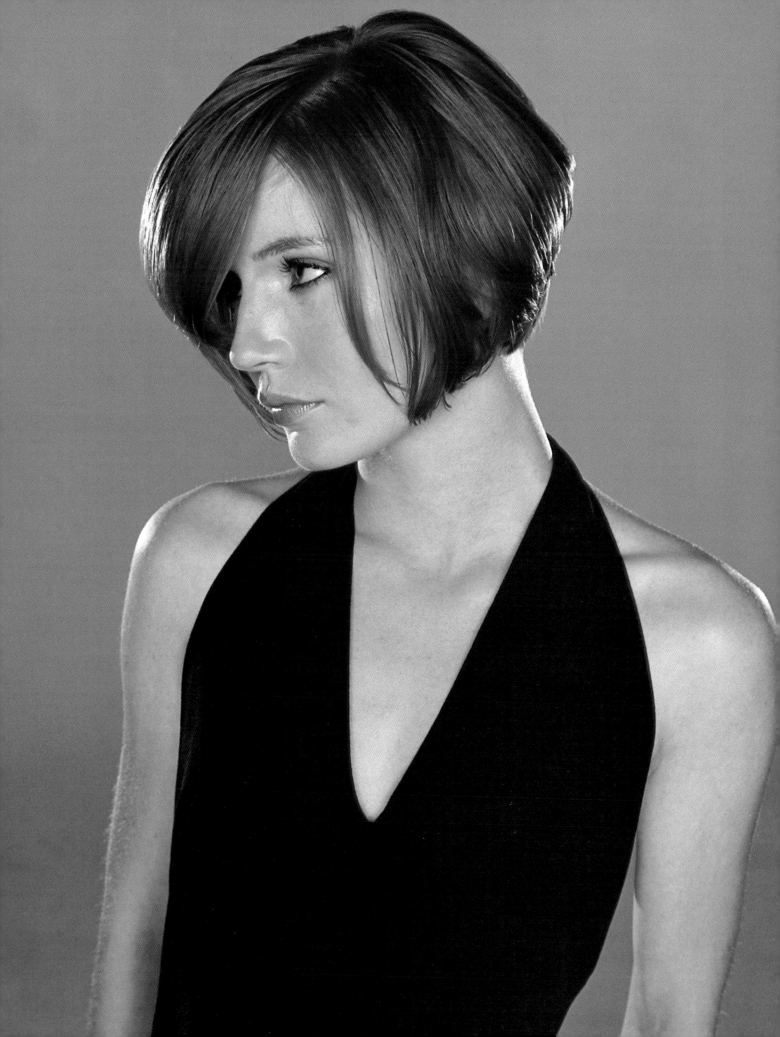

Cutting

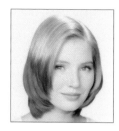

Fine strawberry blonde hair losing its copper sheen with maturity.

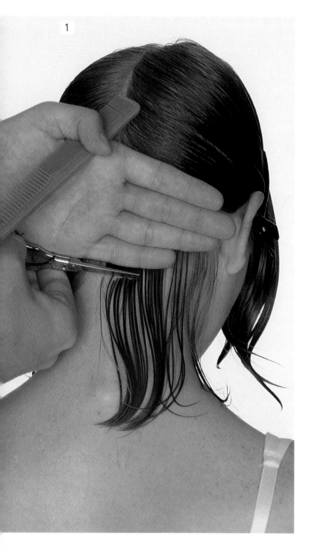

Take your first section horizontally behind the ears, just below the occipital bone. Comb hair until the tension is completely even. Gently press the hair against the skin with either the back of your hand or your fingers and cut a straight line at the nape of the neck.

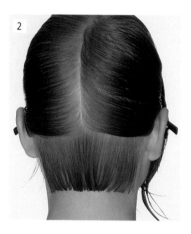

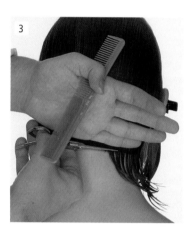

Once you have completed your guide line, continue taking sections in this fashion. Each section should be approximately 2 cm wide. As you work up above the occipital bone, your sections should become diagonal and should not go above the top of the ears. Stop when you reach the crown.

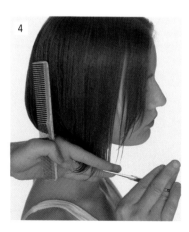

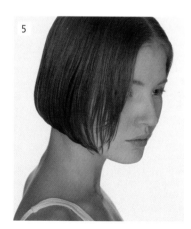

Take a section from the temple to the hair you cut in steps 1 and 2. Comb hair until the tension is even. Hold the hair gently in your fingers and cut, making sure you hold the hair as close to the skin as possible. Work up in this fashion until you reach the centre top. Then do the same on the other side.

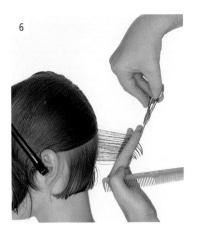

6

You are now ready to start graduating the back. Take a panel from just above the occipital bone to behind the ears, starting at the centre back. Take a vertical section approximately 1 cm wide, pull out at a 45 degree angle and cut. The hair at the nape should still be approximately 3 cm long, so there should be very little cut at the bottom. Be careful not to cut into your guide line, as this will alter the shape of your haircut. As you move across the head towards the ears, you should be pulling each section straight back. Be careful not to over direct back to your original section.

7

Continue to take horizontal panels approximately 5 cm wide. It should take you about 3 panels to work up to the crown. Continue taking vertical sections, at a 45 degree angle, pulling each section straight out from the head. Each panel should blend into the longest part of the previously cut panel. Make sure both sides are cut the same.

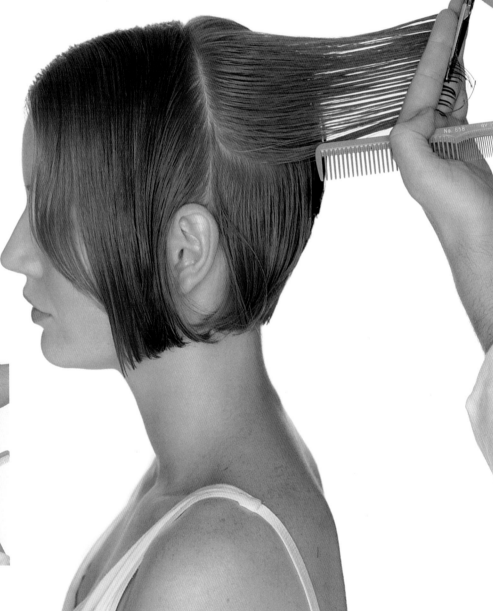

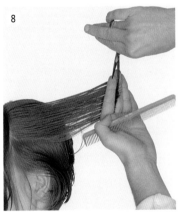

8

Once the back is completed, over direct all the hair in front of the ears back to the graduation you cut in step 7.

Colouring

1

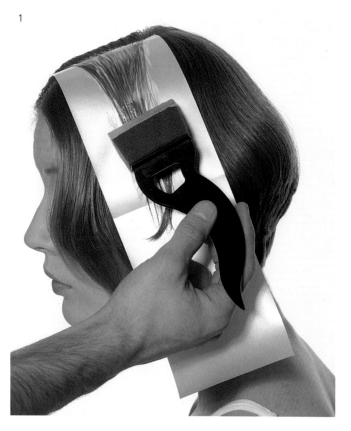

Take a fine slice from the parting and place it over a Colour Wrap. Using a Colour Stroker, apply a barrier cream from the roots down to the ends.

2

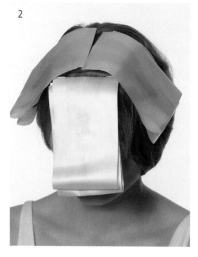

Repeat on the other side of the parting and the fringe area.

3

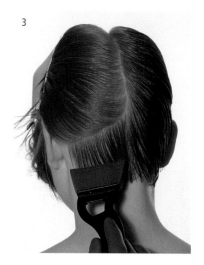

4

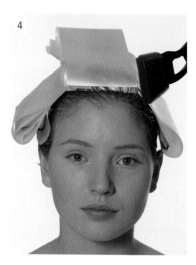

5

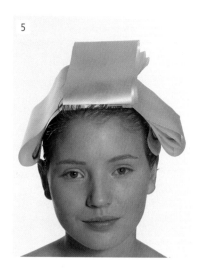

Starting at the nape, apply the semi-permanent colour using the Colour Stroker. Continue this working pattern to cover the rest of the hair.

Colour technique is now complete. Allow to develop under heat/Climazon for 15 minutes. Then rinse hair thoroughly.

PRODUCTS USED

- Wella stain guard
- Color Touch 8/43 Indian Copper mixed in equal parts with Color Touch Developer
- SP 4.V Designing Fluid
- SP 3.E Active Repair Fluid

1

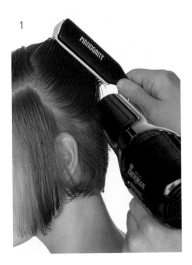

2

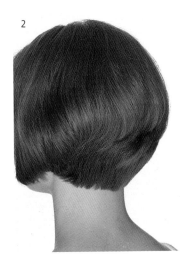

Blow-dry the hair using a Denman classic brush for smooth finish.

Note that there are no heavy weight lines and the graduation has a beautiful bevelled shape.

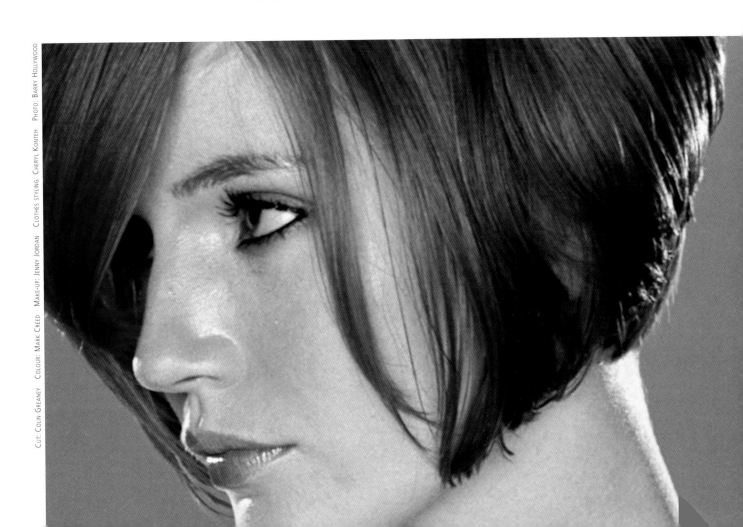

Cut: Colin Greaney   Colour: Mark Creed   Make-up: Jenny Jordan   Clothes styling: Cheryl Konteh   Photo: Barry Hollywood

GRADUATED BOB (2)

Graduated bob with a round bevelled neckline.

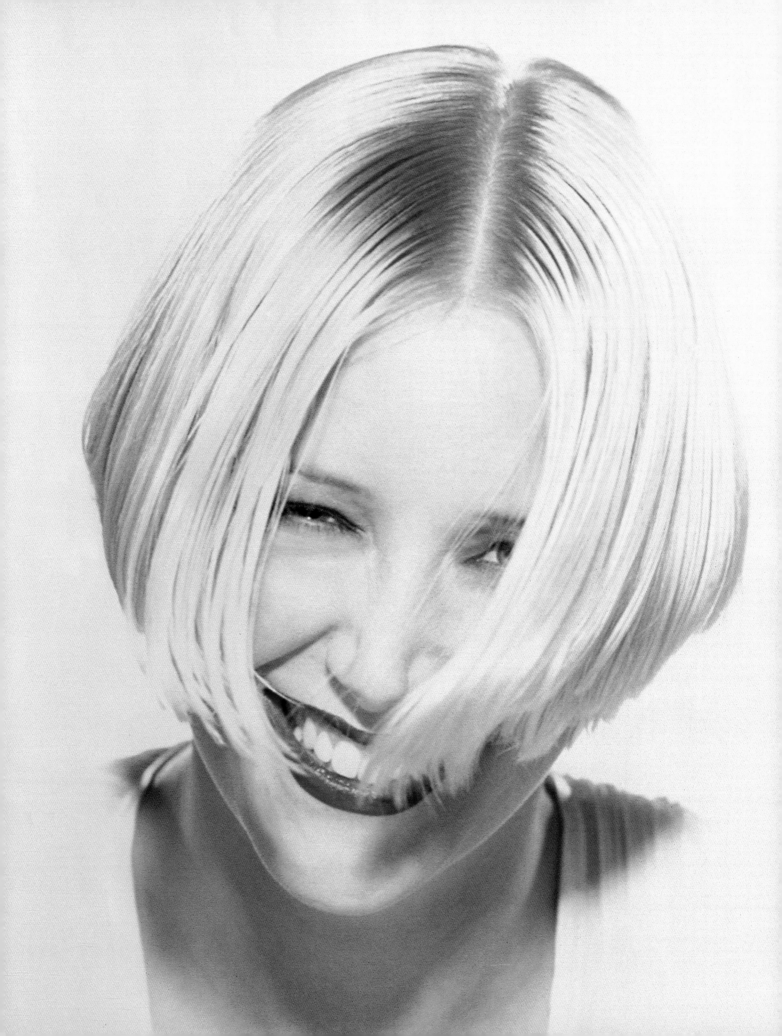

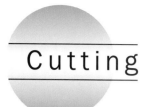

Cutting

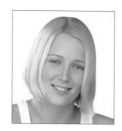

The model's hair was in a grown-out bob shape. She still wanted a bob but with more bounce and swing.

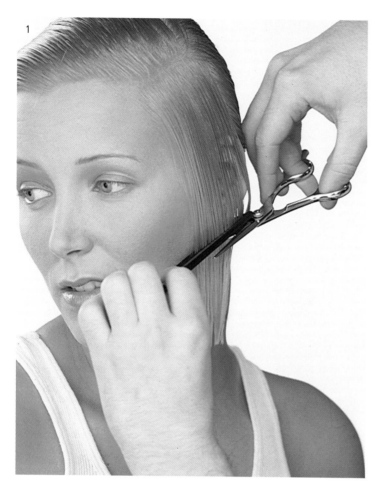

1

The model wanted the sides to be in line with her lips. Start at the side so that you can cut your line on the face to the desired length.

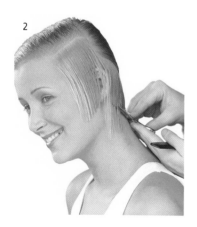

2

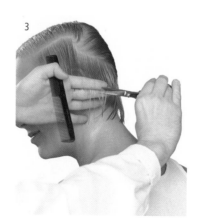

3

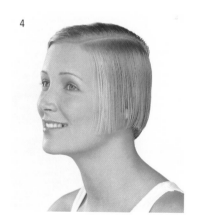

4

The line into the back will create a round neckline. Angle the line downwards into the centre back using the side panel as the guide.

5

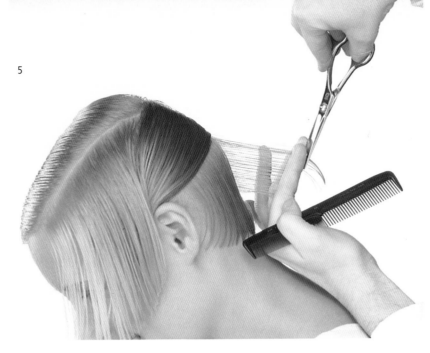

Take your first panel from ear to ear. Take the first section at 45 degrees, continue the section parallel to the head and continue this line into the next panel to the crown.

6

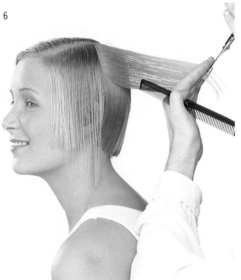

7

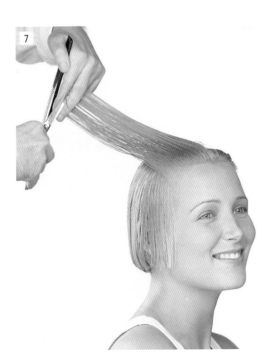

Continue into the sides over directing to the back of the ear.

Finishing

1

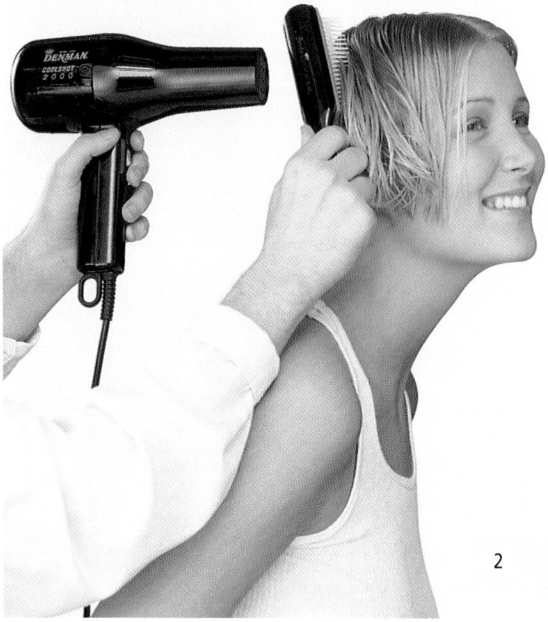

Using a Denman classic brush,
dry the hair section by section.

2

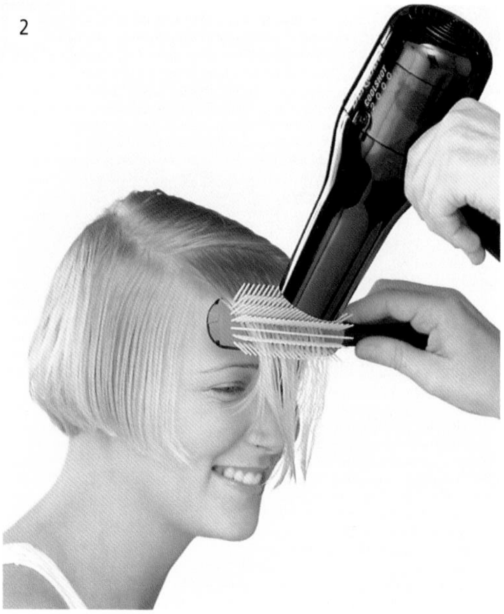

TIP

Make sure you dry the
lengths right the way through
to the ends. If you do not,
the ends will not be neat.

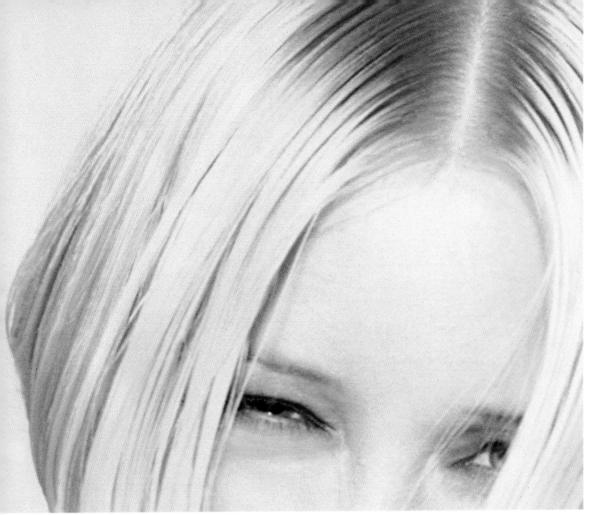

PRODUCTS
USED

• SP 4.V Designing Fluid

• SP 3.E Active Repair
  Fluid

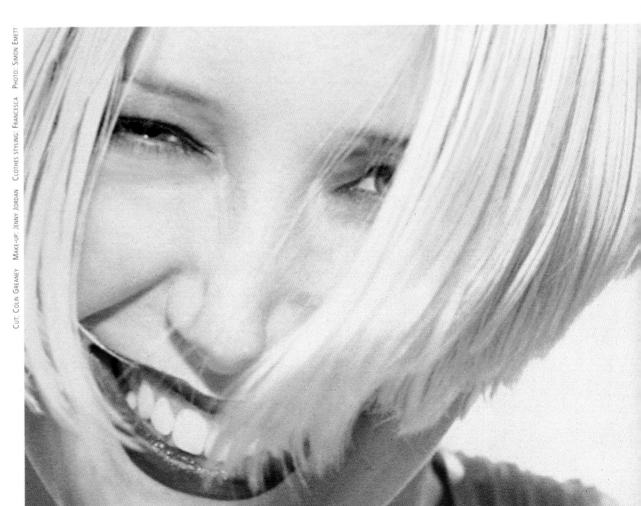

CUT: COLIN GREANEY   MAKE-UP: JENNY JORDAN   CLOTHES STYLING: FRANCESCA   PHOTO: SIMON EMETT

ONE LENGTH BOB
WITH A FRINGE

Precision-cut outline complemented

by a square-cut fringe.

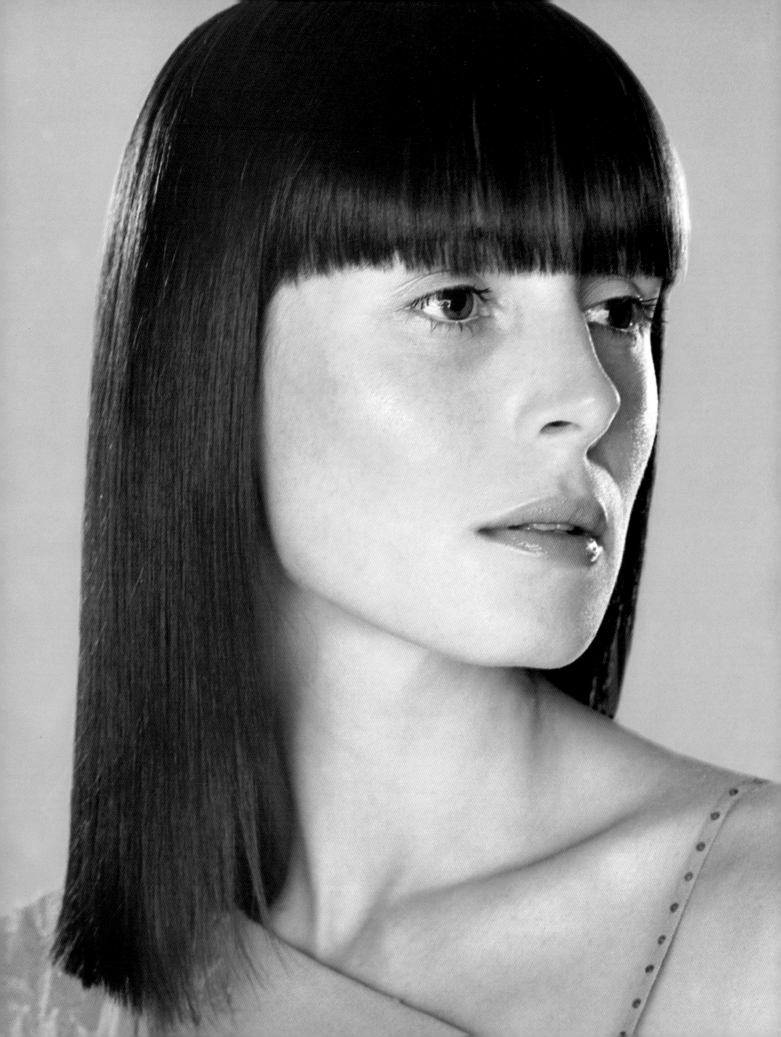

Colouring

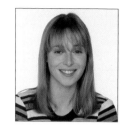

The model's hair is medium fine and was heavily highlighted. The model wanted darker, warm shiny hair. The cut will have a sharp square-cut fringe and a square blunt-cut outline.

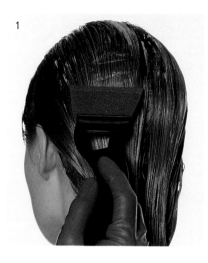

Apply a pre-pigmentation rinse to the whole head using a Colour Stroker. Leave to develop for 5 minutes under heat/Climazon. Rinse and dry with a hairdryer.

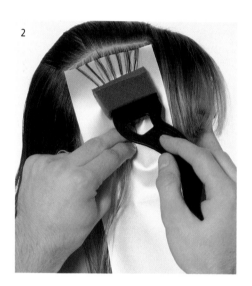

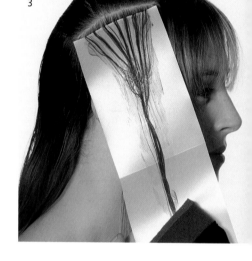

Take a section 2 cm under the parting and place a fine woven mesh on a Colour Wrap. Apply the colour with a Colour Stroker.

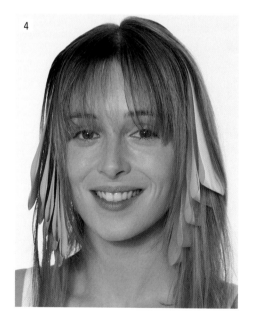

Finished sections. Note only the underneath layer has been coloured using the Colour Wraps.

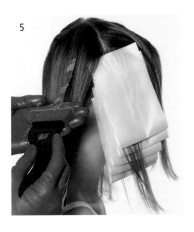

5

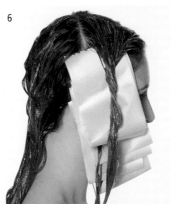

6

Use a Colour Stroker to apply the target shade to the middle lengths and ends, starting 4 cm from the scalp. Leave to develop for 10 minutes under heat/Climazon.

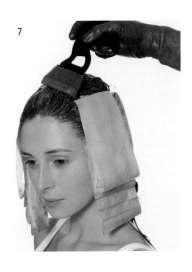

7

Mix fresh colour of the same shade and apply to root area. Develop for a further 10 minutes under heat/Climazon. When development is complete, rinse, shampoo and condition as normal.

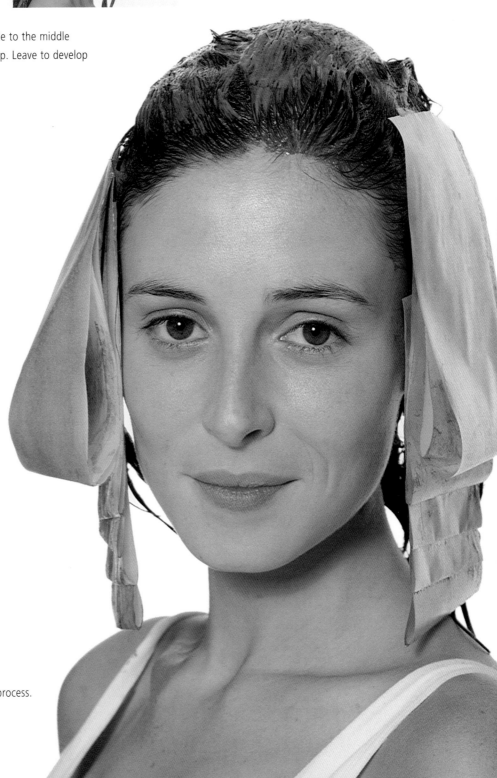

8

Colour finished. Allow to process.

Cutting

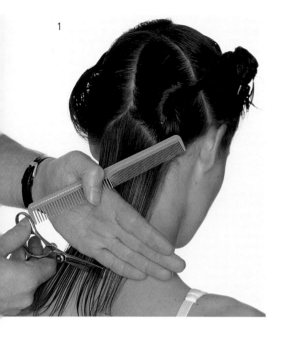

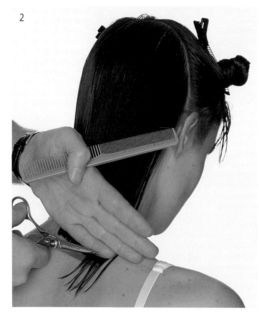

Section the hair parallel to the hairline. From the centre back, stretching the hair firmly and following the natural fall, cut a slightly inverted line. Continue this on both sides up to the crown and to the centre top of the ear.

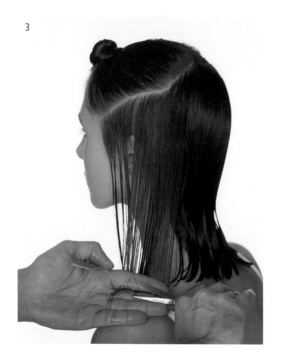

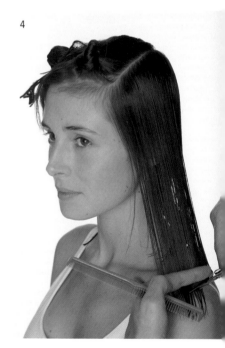

Follow the line through into the sides, allowing the section to relax slightly over the ear to allow for the ear lifting the outline. Continue this line on both sides up to a centre parting.

5

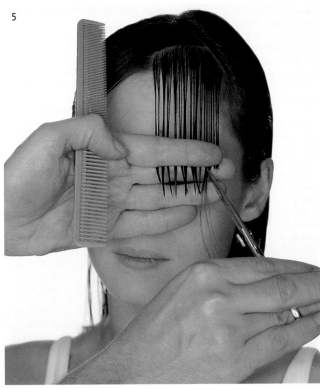

Separate a triangular section from temple to temple (the head shape determines the heaviness of the fringe). Point cutting the fringe gives a naturalistic effect. Continue this square line and point technique on each section.

6

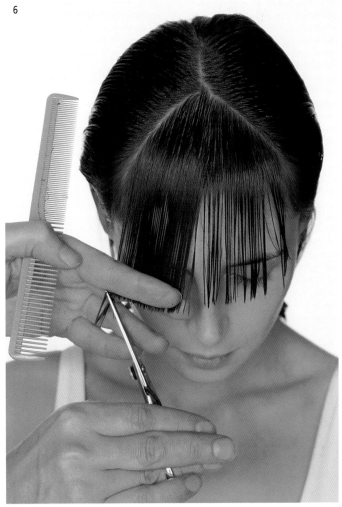

Finishing

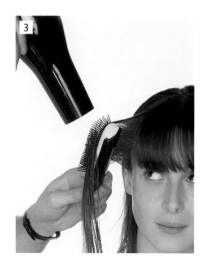

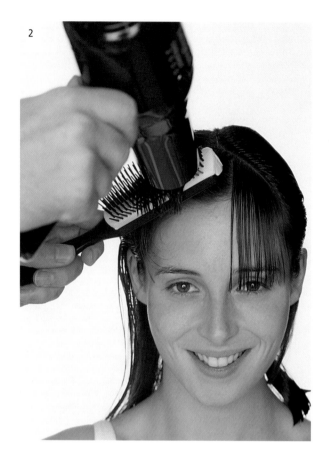

Apply a blow-drying lotion then start blow-drying at the fringe – this is the shortest hair and needs to be dried first, before it dries. This also allows your client to get an idea of the look.

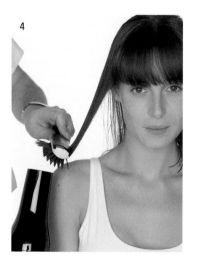

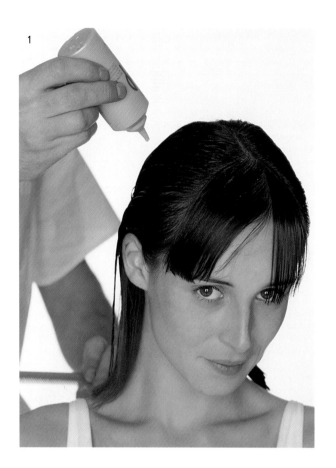

It is important to get a very straight finish. Using a Denman classic brush, lift the hair at the root and follow down the length of the hair with the hairdryer to keep all stray ends smooth, creating finish and shine. When you get to the end of the section, reverse your brush position. This will give the required straightness to fall on the shoulder line.

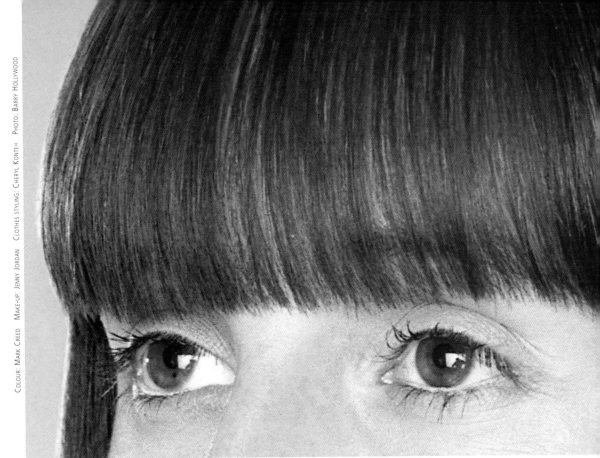

COLOUR: MARK CREED   MAKE-UP: JENNY JORDAN   CLOTHES STYLING: CHERYL KONTEH   PHOTO: BARRY HOLYWOOD

A simple effective long bob with superb shine and finish, the hair gleaming with health and beauty.

PRODUCTS USED

- Koleston Perfect 8/43 Celtic Copper mixed with 12% Welloxon Perfect Creme Developer

- Koleston Perfect 6/75 Rich Heather mixed with 12% Welloxon Perfect Creme Developer

- SP 4.V Designing Fluid

- SP 3.E Active Repair Fluid

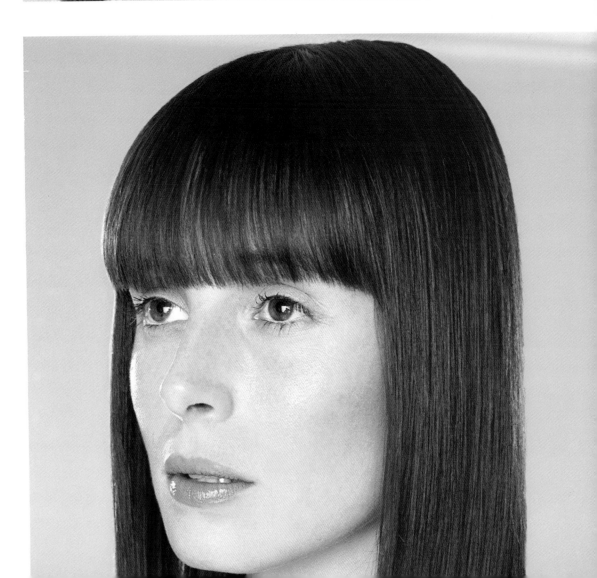

CLASSIC LONG LAYERS

Long layers creating a loose natural shape.

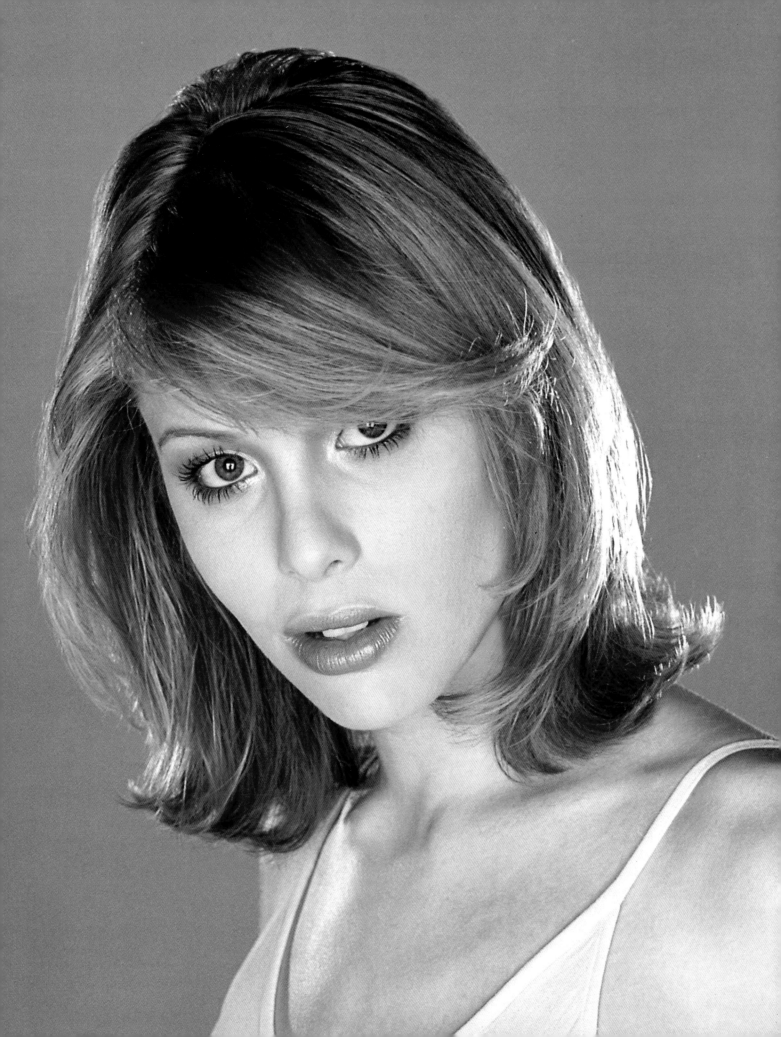

Cutting

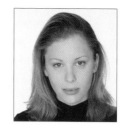

The model's hair was approximately the desired overall length at the back but she required more shape around the face. The outline length at the back is cut in the same way as the classic shoulder length bob (see page 42), then the outline shape is created around the face. The hair may be dressed for greater volume.

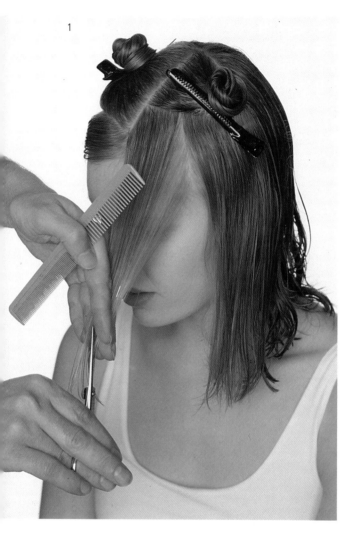

1

Starting from a centre parting, cut a line from the corner of the eye to meet the corner of the square bob-shaped back, and continue this on both sides until your sectioning reaches the crown.

TIP

Take care that the head is in the same position and each section is held out at the same angle to the head.

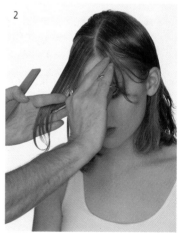

2

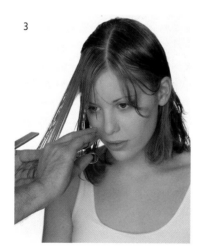

3

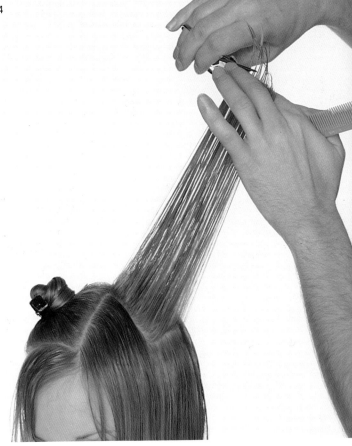

TIP

Maintain even tension throughout.

Lifting the top sections (everything above the temple line), layer them away to a line as shown. This layering will give you total versatility when dressing the hair.

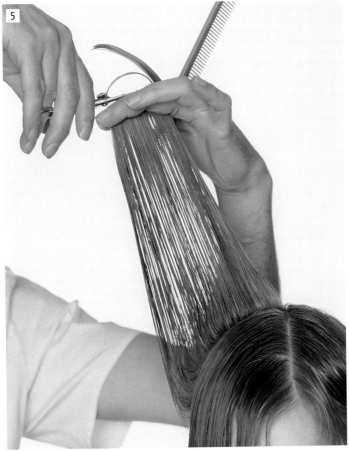

5

Colouring

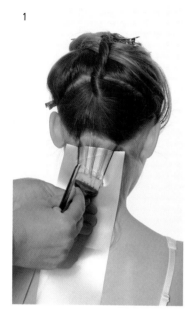

1

Starting at the nape of the neck, take a section 1 cm in depth and slightly narrower than the Colour Wrap. Weave out a fine section and apply the mid-tone colour.

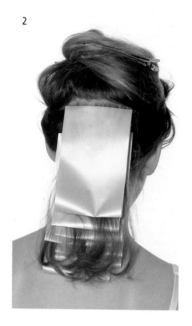

2

Continue to a little way above the occipital bone, alternating your colours and making sure you keep the weave even.

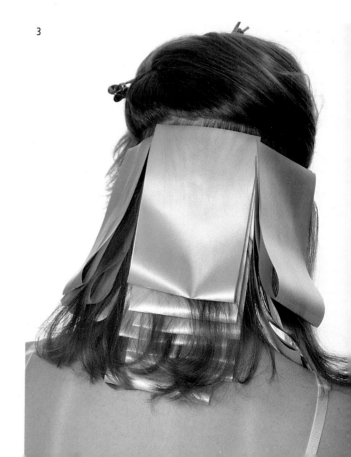

3

Taking sections on each side of your first packets, repeat to the same level.

4

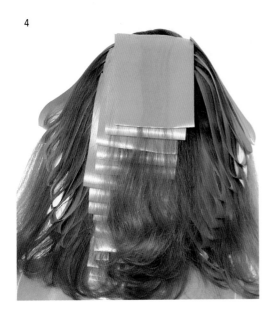

Return to the centre panel and continue up to the crown, making sure you end on your lightest colour at the top.

5

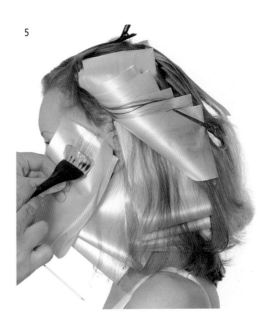

Moving to the side temple area, take your section at a 45 degree angle to the face and continue up to the ear level. From that point return the sections to the horizontal.

6

To improve the look of the hair which contained old colour, a tone on tone semi-permanent was applied between the packets and the whole head processed for 20 minutes.

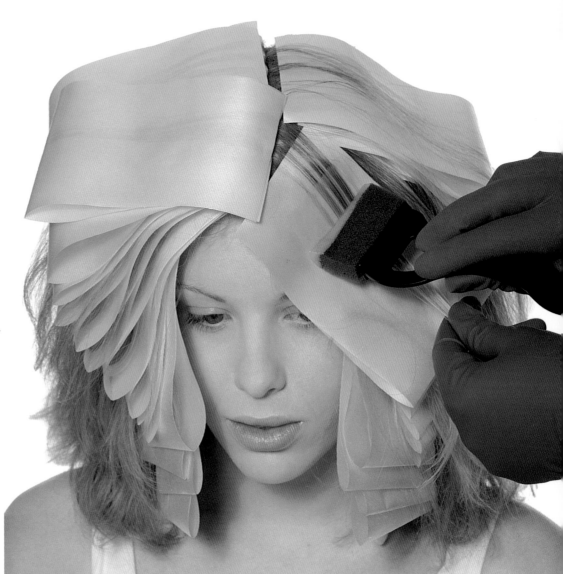

Finishing

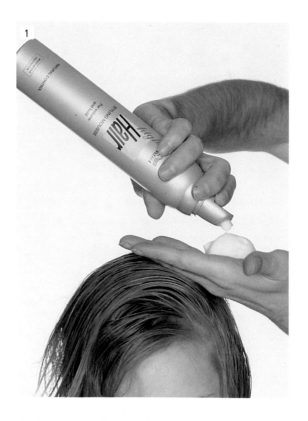

Apply mousse evenly to wet hair.

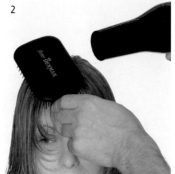

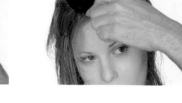

Dry the hair using a paddle brush, brushing backwards and forwards across the centre parting to create root lift.

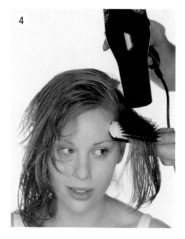

When the hair is half dry, use a classic brush, guiding each section in the desired direction for the finished look.

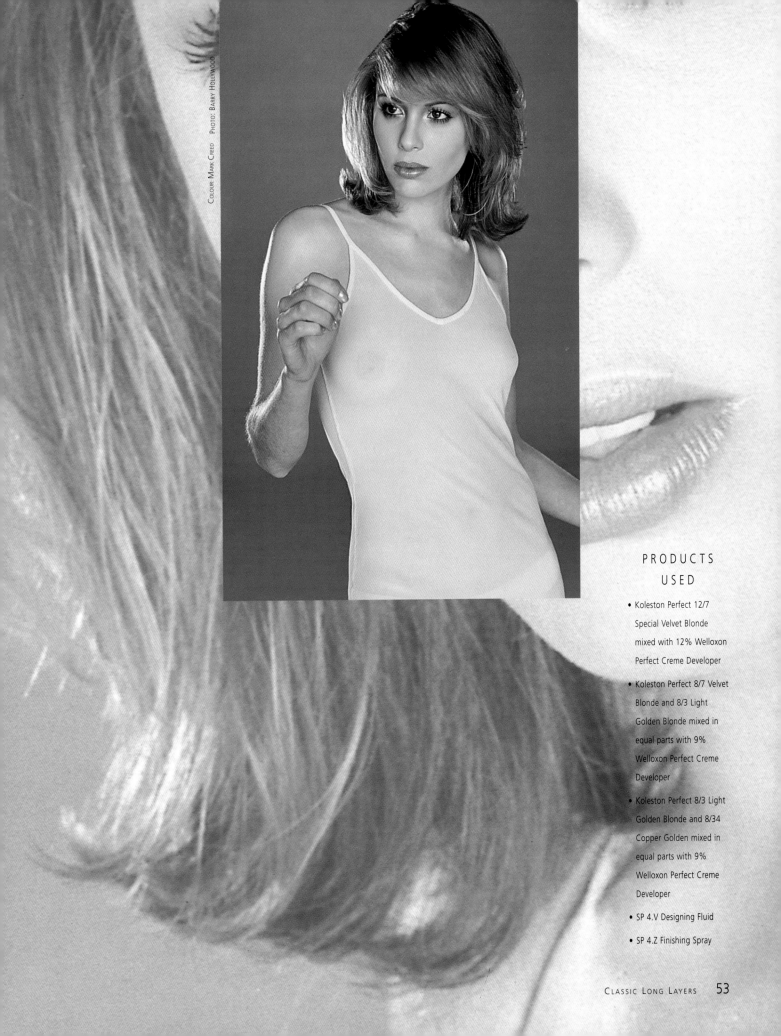

PRODUCTS USED

- Koleston Perfect 12/7 Special Velvet Blonde mixed with 12% Welloxon Perfect Creme Developer

- Koleston Perfect 8/7 Velvet Blonde and 8/3 Light Golden Blonde mixed in equal parts with 9% Welloxon Perfect Creme Developer

- Koleston Perfect 8/3 Light Golden Blonde and 8/34 Copper Golden mixed in equal parts with 9% Welloxon Perfect Creme Developer

- SP 4.V Designing Fluid

- SP 4.Z Finishing Spray

CLASSIC SHORT LAYERS

Short layered shape with texture
throughout the interior.

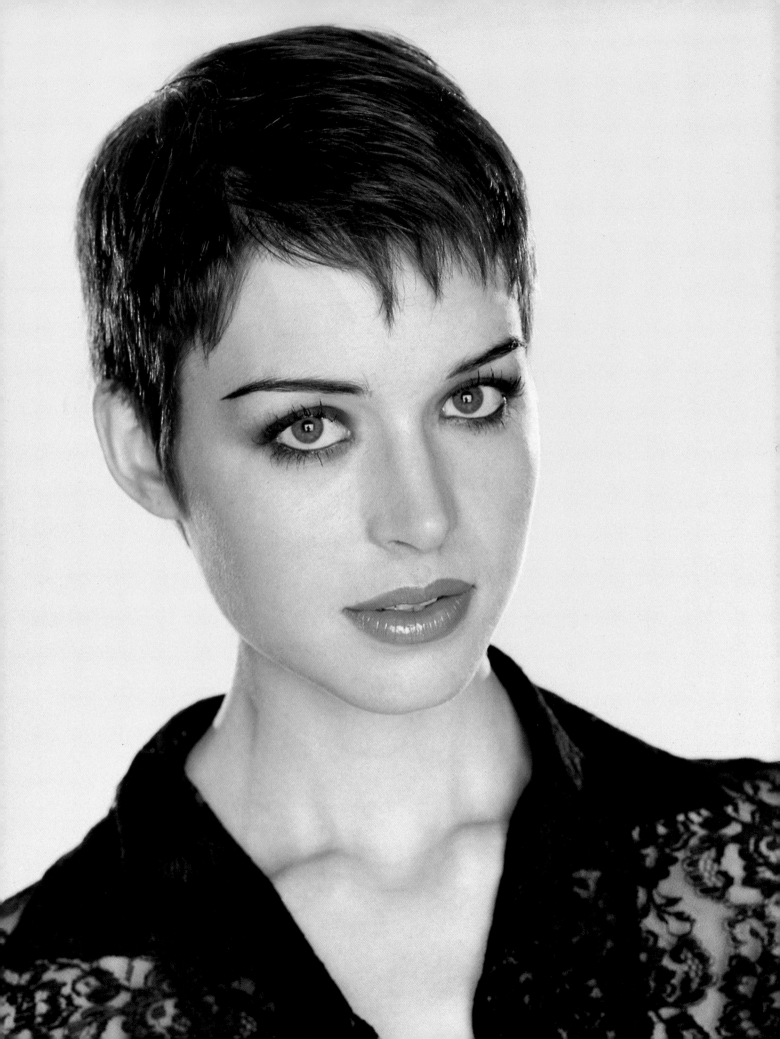

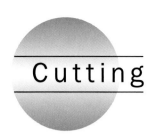

Cutting

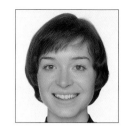

The model's hair had been cut into a shortish layered rounded shape with no particular definition. After consultation, the model decided to have a soft textured crop.

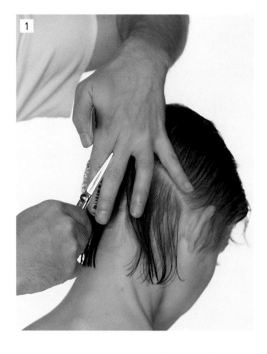

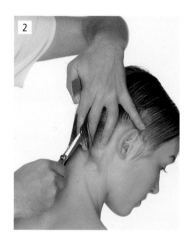

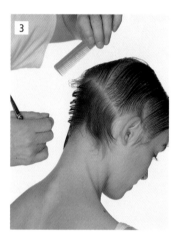

Start the cut at the centre back. Take a section underneath the occipital bone and cut vertically into the nape (approximately 2 cm long). Keeping the section parallel to the head shape, continue all the way across the back.

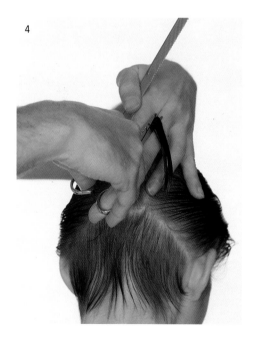

Continue your line up to the crown, keeping your line straight to your original. This creates a length of about 4 cm at the crown.

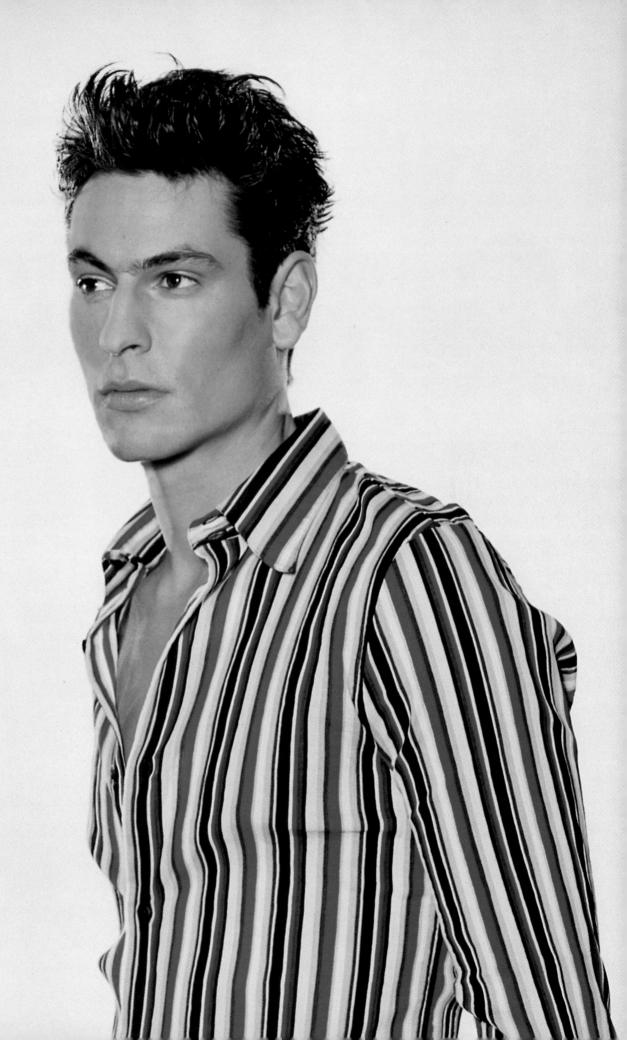

Cutting

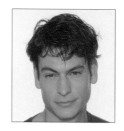

The model's hair had grown out from his previous haircut and had become too bulky at the sides. After consultation we agreed on a shorter, sharper but still textured image.

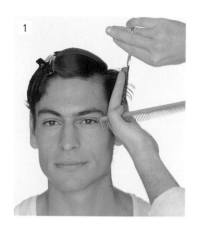

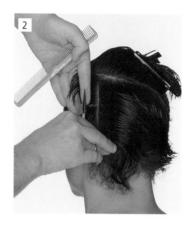

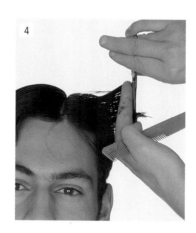

Section off the first panel from the temple to just below the crown. Take your first section at the temples and cut vertically, angling your fingers in towards the ear. The hair should be approximately 2 cm long at the top of the section and approximately 1 cm long at the bottom. Repeat on opposite side.

Continue in this fashion, but as you move round the head to behind the ears, continue the sections down to the nape area. Repeat on opposite side.

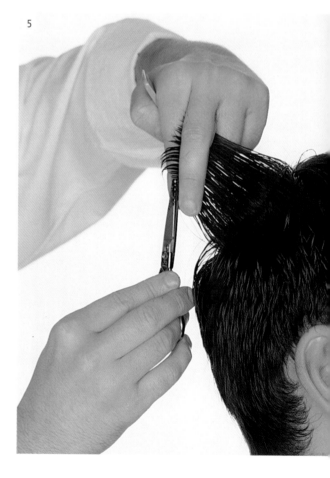

Take your next panel just below a centre parting around to the centre back, just below the crown. Continue taking vertical sections, using the previously cut hair underneath as your guide line. Start at the temple and make sure your section stays parallel to the head, as this will achieve a gradual build up of weight around the crown. Move around the head to the centre back and repeat on the other side.

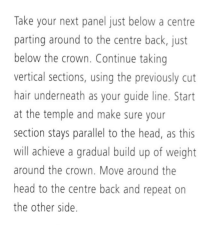

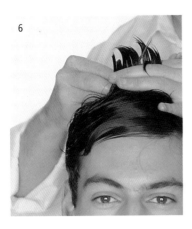

6

You will now be left with the centre top panel left uncut. To achieve the desired textured look, take horizontal sections across the top of the head. Starting at the crown, cut into the hair at different lengths. Take care not to cut the hair too short as this will make the rest of the haircut appear unbalanced. Continue in this manner towards the front of the head.

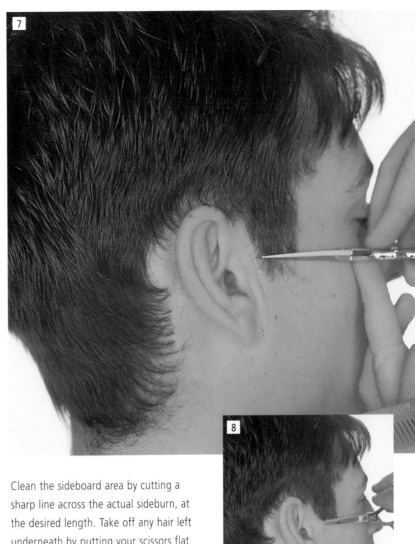

7

Clean the sideboard area by cutting a sharp line across the actual sideburn, at the desired length. Take off any hair left underneath by putting your scissors flat against the skin and cutting. It is important to keep the movement of your scissors as flowing as possible.

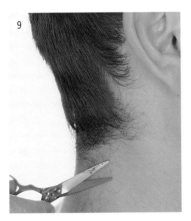

9

Use the same technique to take off fuzzy hair at the nape.

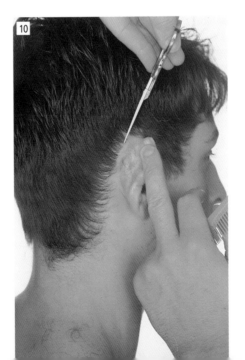

10

Take off any untidy hair around the ears by gently pulling the ear down and cutting a sharp line.

Finishing

1

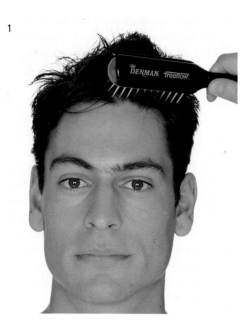

Blow-dry using a Denman vent brush to achieve texture.

2

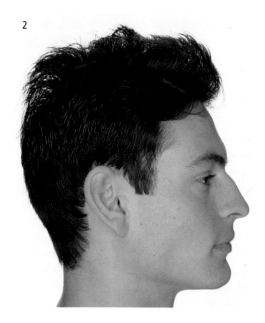

You should have no weight lines anywhere in the haircut, and it should hug the natural shape of the head.

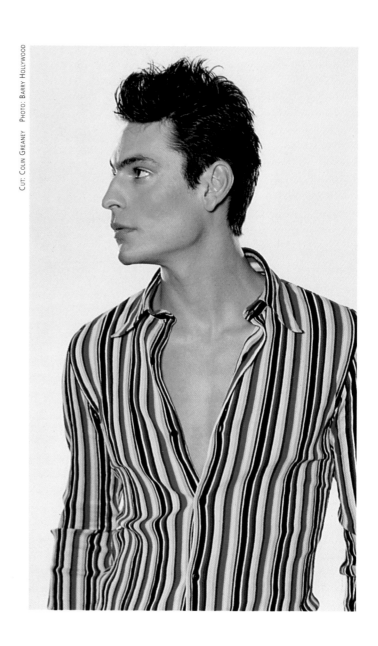

CUT: COLIN GREANEY   PHOTO: BARRY HOLLYWOOD

PRODUCTS
USED

• SP 3.S Restructuring
Complex with Liquid Hair

• High Hair Shine Mousse
Pomade

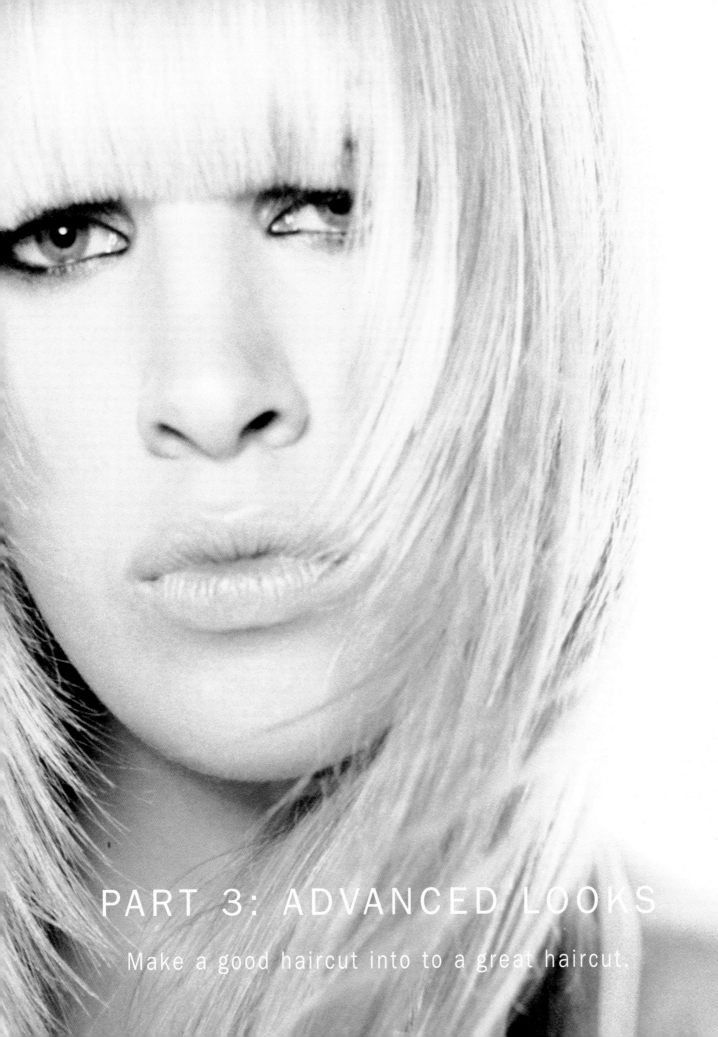

PART 3: ADVANCED LOOKS

Make a good haircut into to a great haircut.

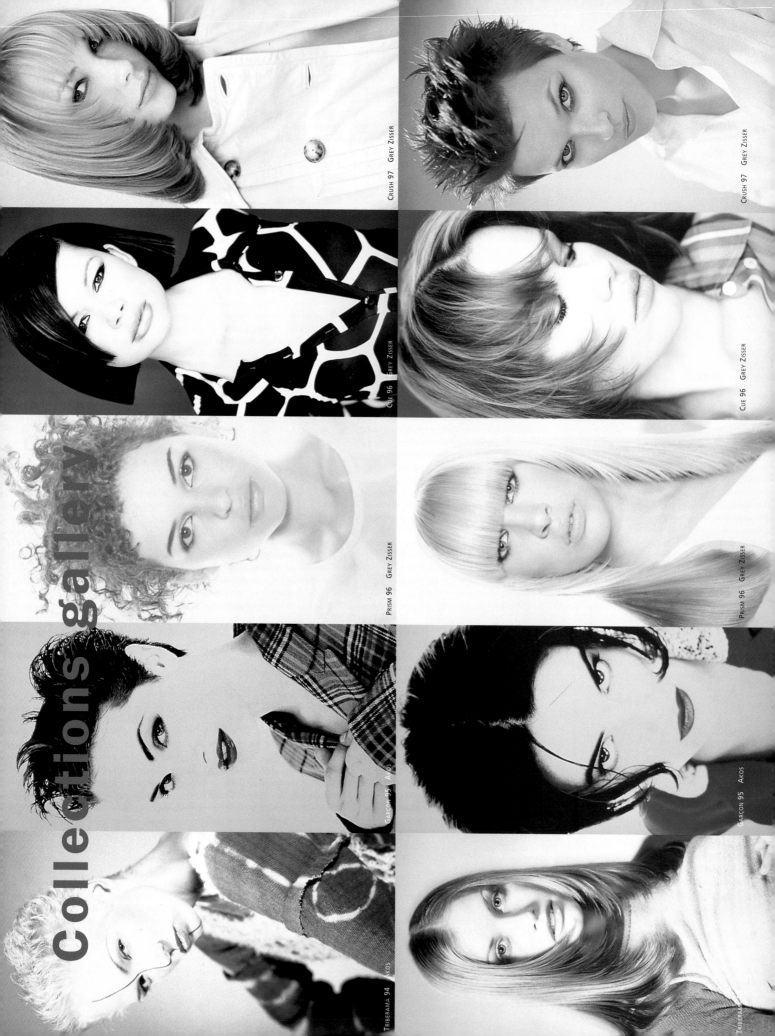

collections gallery

CRUSH 97   GREY ZISSER

CRUSH 97   GREY ZISSER

CUE 96   GREY ZISSER

CUE 96   GREY ZISSER

PRISM 96   GREY ZISSER

PRISM 96   GREY ZISSER

GARÇON 95   AKOS

GARÇON 95   AKOS

TRIBERAMA 94   AKOS

TRIBERAMA

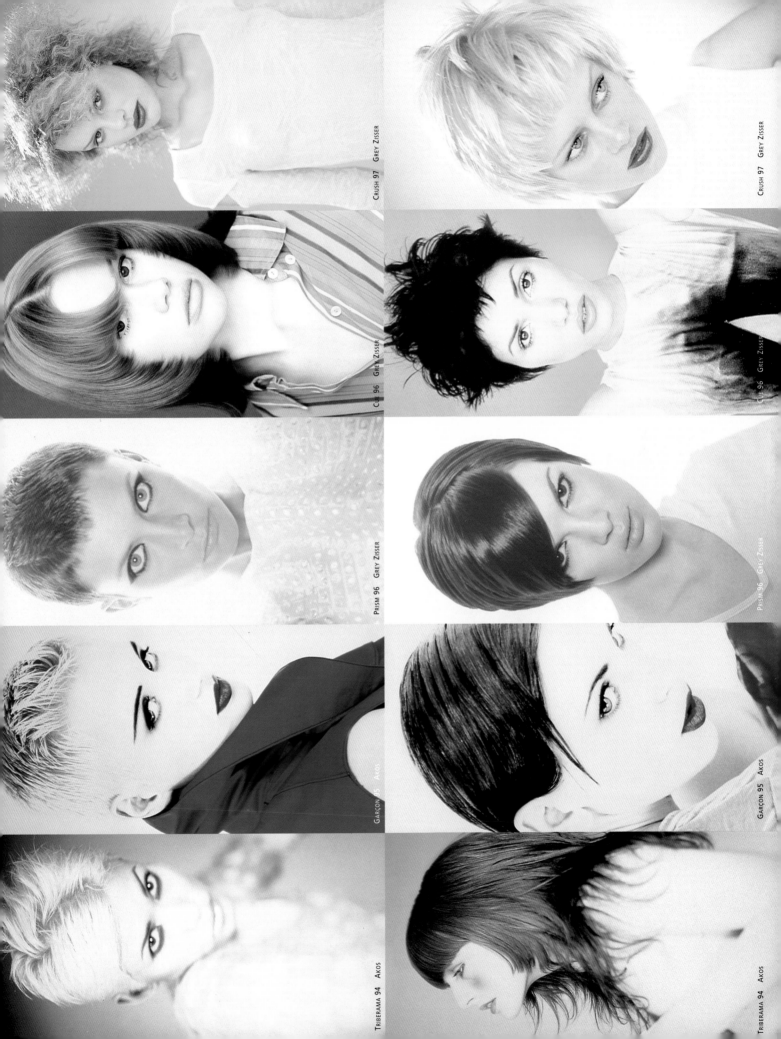

CRUSH 97 GREY ZISSER

CRUSH 97 GREY ZISSER

CUE 96 GREY ZISSER

CUE 96 GREY ZISSER

PRISM 96 GREY ZISSER

PRISM 96 GREY ZISSER

GARÇON 95 AKOS

GARÇON 95 AKOS

TRIBERAMA 94 AKOS

TRIBERAMA 94 AKOS

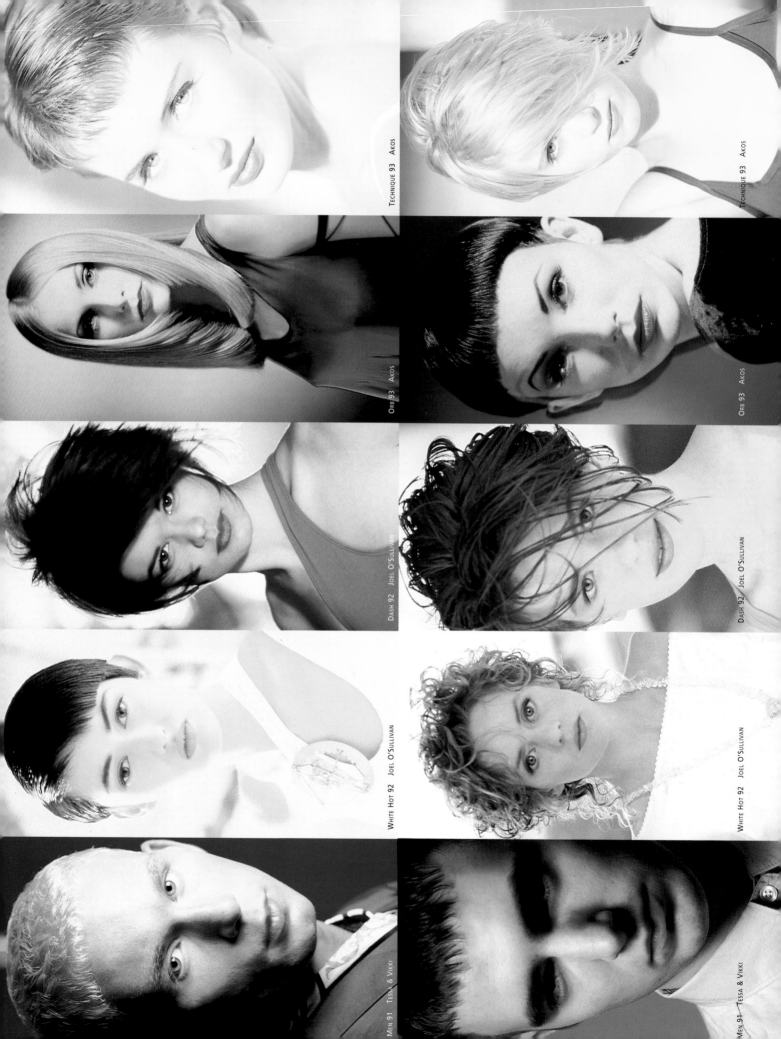

TECHNIQUE 93   AKOS

TECHNIQUE 93   AKOS

ORB 93   AKOS

ORB 93   AKOS

DASH 92   JOEL O'SULLIVAN

DASH 92   JOEL O'SULLIVAN

WHITE HOT 92   JOEL O'SULLIVAN

WHITE HOT 92   JOEL O'SULLIVAN

MEN 91   TESSA & VIKKI

MEN 91   TESSA & VIKKI

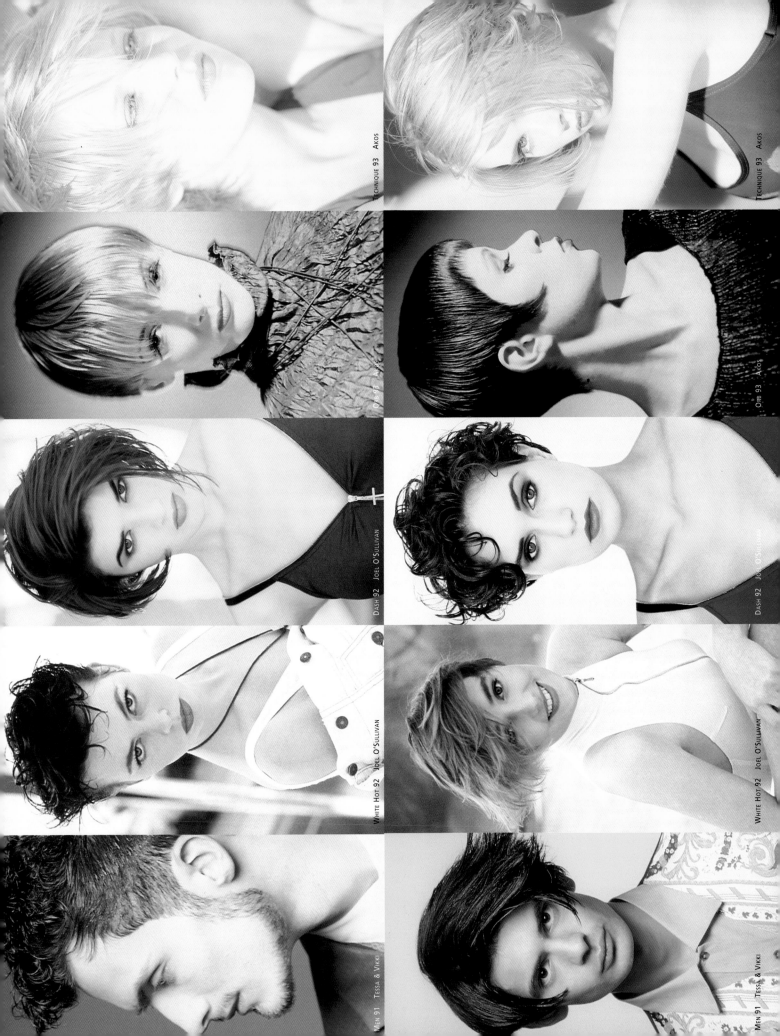

TECHNIQUE 93   AKOS

TECHNIQUE 93   AKOS

ORB 93   AKOS

ORB 93   AKOS

DASH 92   JOEL O'SULLIVAN

DASH 92   JOEL O'SULLIVAN

WHITE HOT 92   JOEL O'SULLIVAN

WHITE HOT 92   JOEL O'SULLIVAN

MEN 91   TESSA & VIKKI

MEN 91   TESSA & VIKKI

Fringes

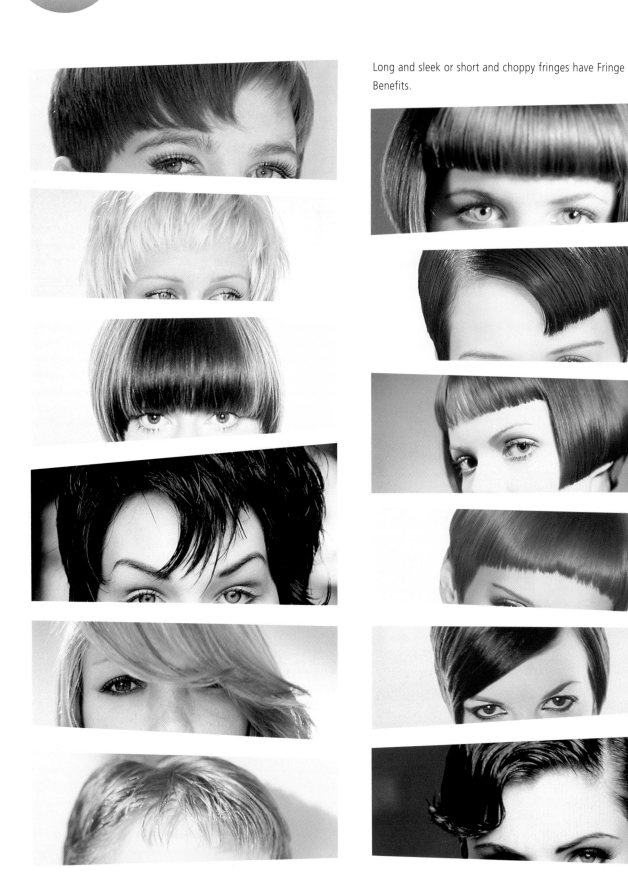

Long and sleek or short and choppy fringes have Fringe Benefits.

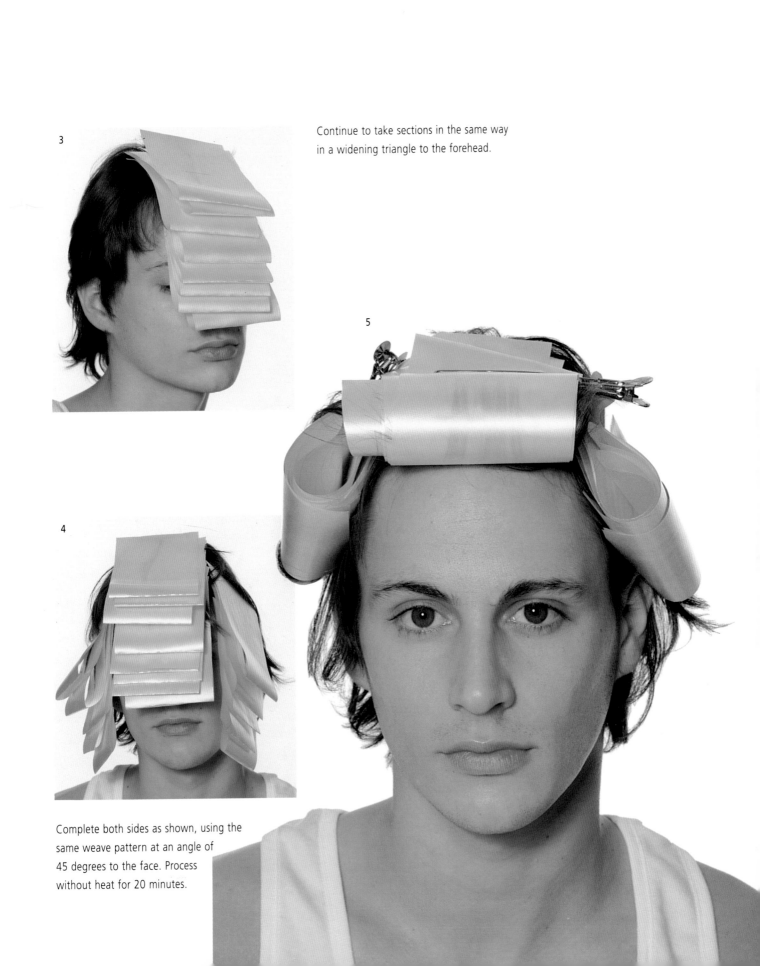

3

Continue to take sections in the same way
in a widening triangle to the forehead.

5

4

Complete both sides as shown, using the
same weave pattern at an angle of
45 degrees to the face. Process
without heat for 20 minutes.

Finishing

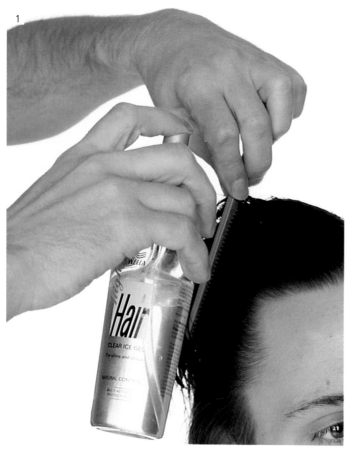

Apply gel evenly to wet hair. Using your fingers like a claw, lift the hair up and away creating lots of root lift during the drying.

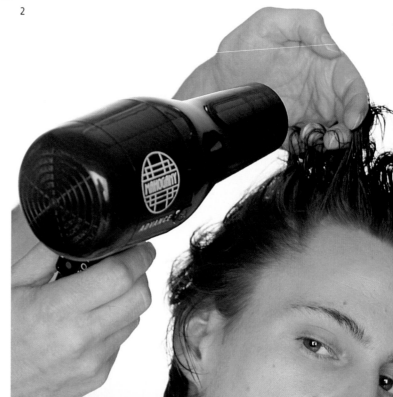

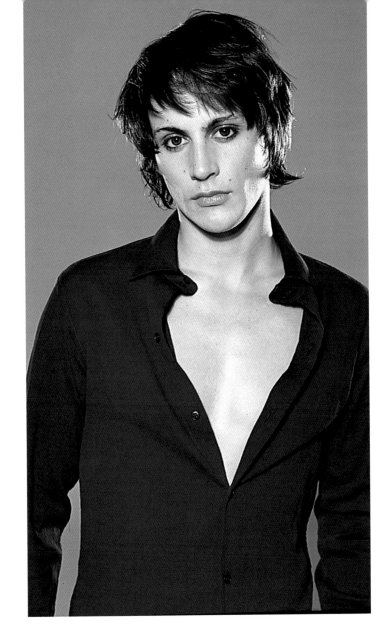

COLOUR MARK CREED PHOTO: BARRY HOLLYWOOD

PRODUCTS USED

- Koleston Perfect 6/3 Dark Golden Blonde mixed with 6% Welloxon Perfect Creme Developer

- Koleston Perfect 8/73 Golden Sand mixed with 9% Welloxon Perfect Creme Developer

- Color Touch 6/7 Persimmon mixed in equal parts with Color Touch Developer

- SP 4.Y Defining Gel

- SP 4.Z Finishing Spray

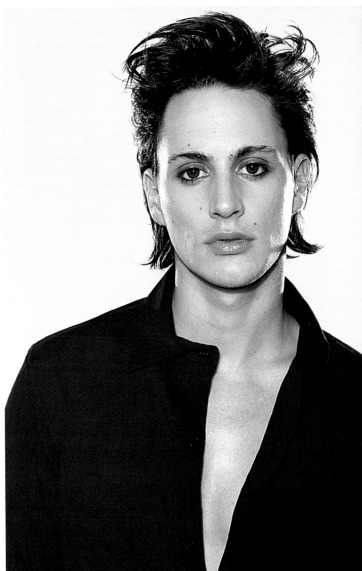

TEXTURED HORIZONTAL SECTIONING TECHNIQUE

Freefall soft geometric look.

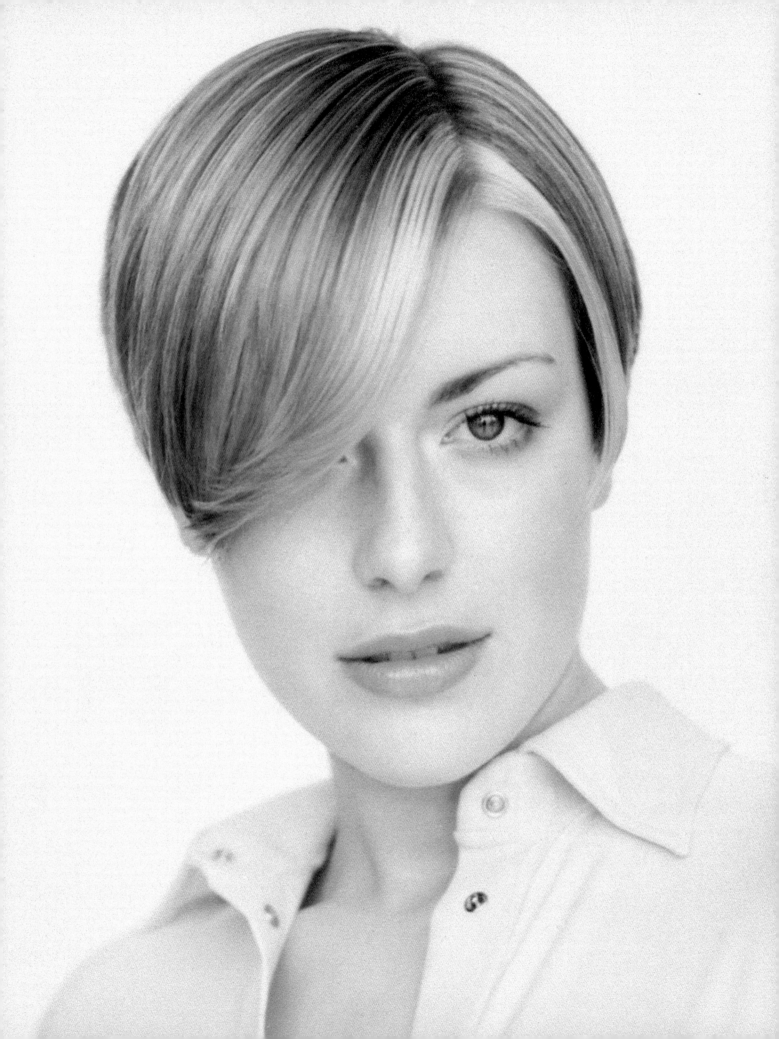

Colouring

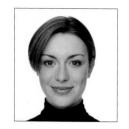

The model's hair had been cut into a short bob shape but she wanted a look which would still be worn smooth but with a looser textured feel and golden sunny colour.

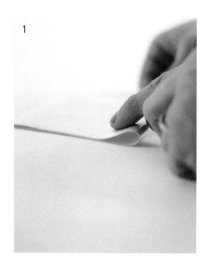

Take approximately 12 Colour Wraps at a time and prefold them. This will make it easier to fold them with precision when they are placed in the hair.

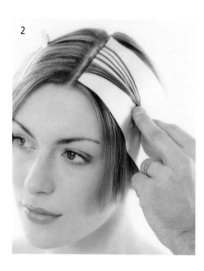

Weave a band 1 cm back from the hairline followed by four individual highlights into the first section.

TIP

Seal the folded Colour Wrap by pressing it with your comb.

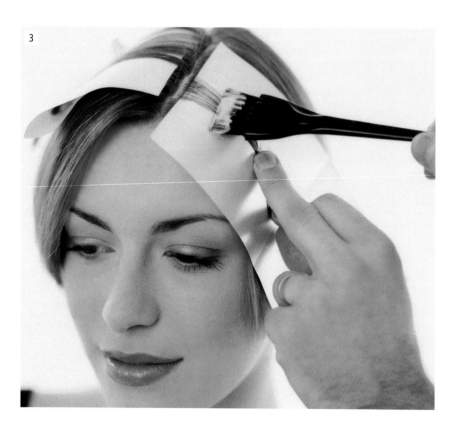

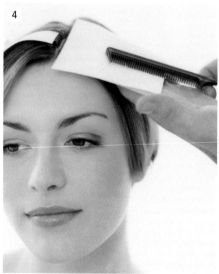

For the next section, take only a band. Place in Colour Wrap as for previous section.

Repeat steps 1–3 on the opposite side.

5

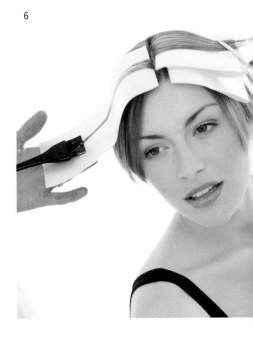

6

7

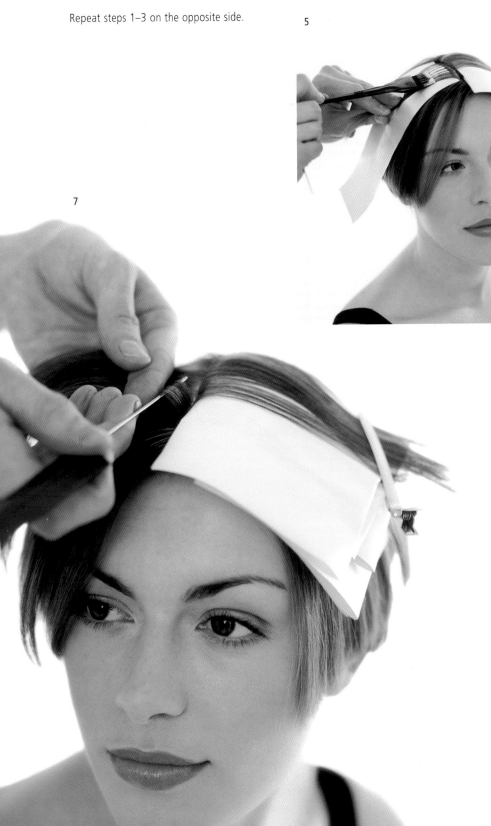

Cutting

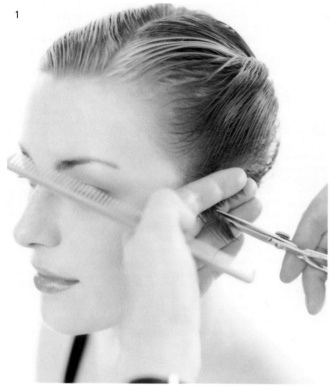

1

Start the cut on the side. Lift the first section at 45 degrees to the side of the head and cut short triangular lines into the edge. Continue this technique up to the centre.

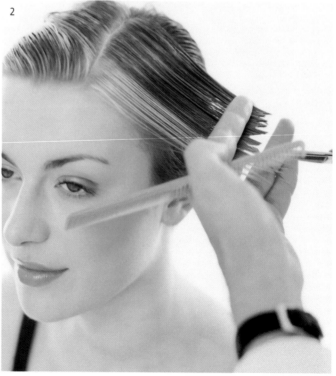

2

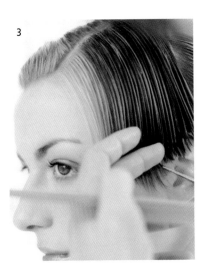

3

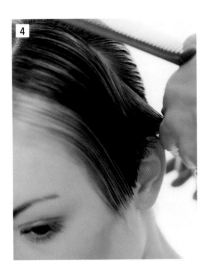

4

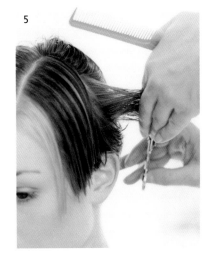

5

The outline is cleaned up still using the same technique.

Using the original line as a guide, continue graduating the hair into the nape.

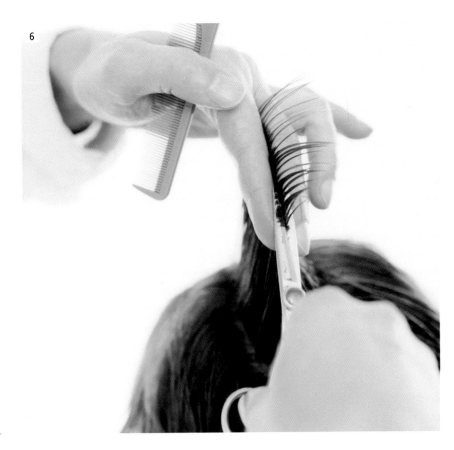

6

As you get to the back of the head, lift the hair to 90 degrees to keep it parallel with the head.

7

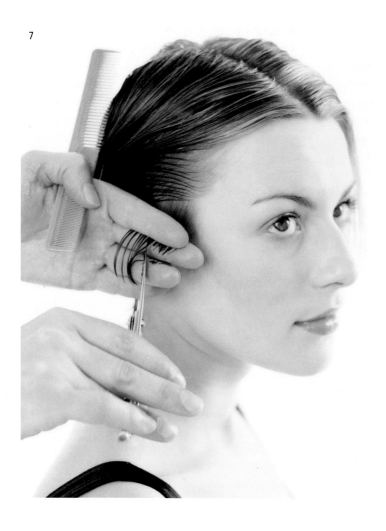

Follow the same technique on the opposite side.

8

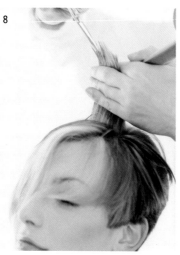

9

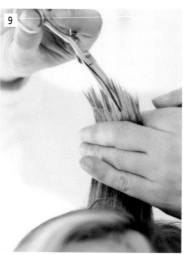

Connect the line across the top and then cut V-shapes into the lengths to create your texture.

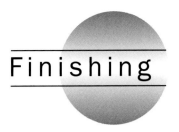

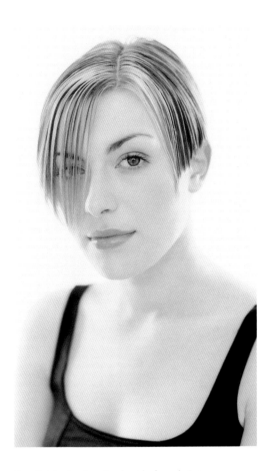

The finished cut and colour before drying.

PRODUCTS USED

- Koleston Perfect 10/3 Light Golden Blonde mixed with 12% Welloxon Perfect Creme Developer

- SP 3.S Restructuring Complex with Liquid Hair

- High Hair Shine Mousse Pomade

- SP 4.Z Finishing Spray

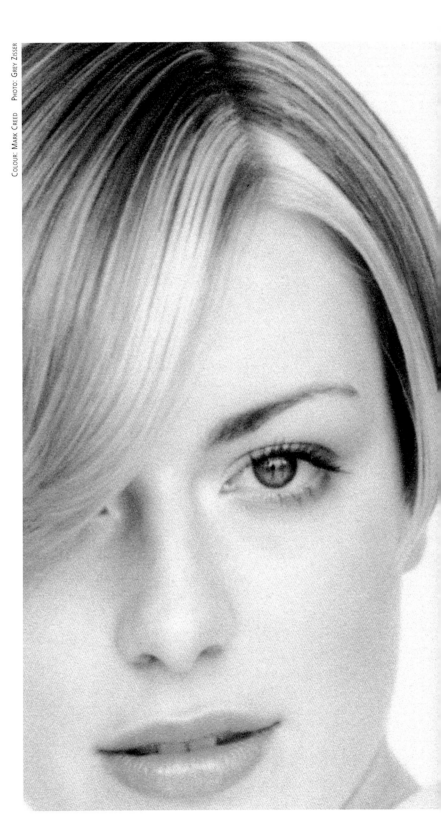

COLOUR: MARK CREED   PHOTO: GREY ZISSER

ASYMMETRIC CUT

Controlled asymmetric shape.

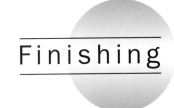

Blow-dry and dress the hair.

PRODUCTS USED

- Koleston Perfect 12/03 Special Beige Blonde (in Colour Wraps)

- Koleston Perfect 6/3 Dark Golden Blonde and 5/4 Deep Autumn Chestnut mixed in equal parts with 6% Welloxon Perfect Creme Developer (full head colour)

- SP 1.8 Colour Vitalising Cleanser

- SP 3.8 Colour Saver

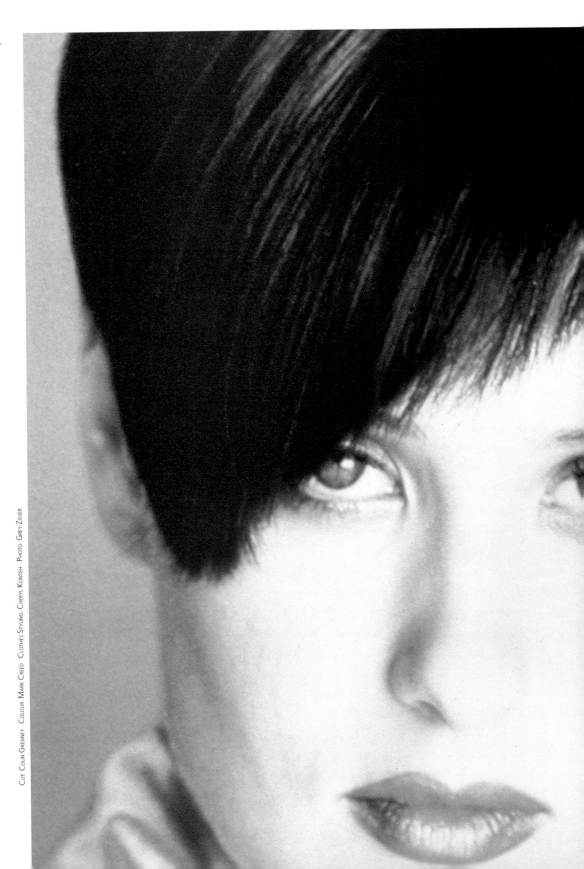

CUT: COLIN GREANEY COLOUR: MARK CREED CLOTHES STYLING: CHERYL KONTEH PHOTO: GREY ZISSER

FEATHERING TECHNIQUE

Heavy square-cut fringe working into
long feathered layers.

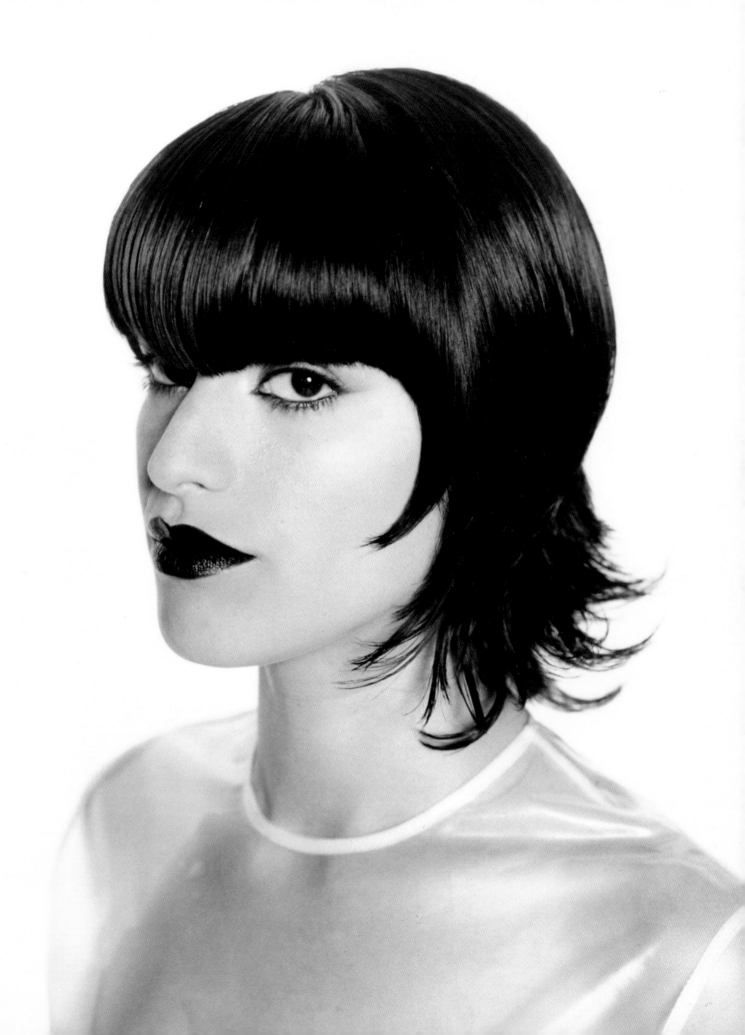

Cutting

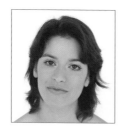

The model wanted a very feathery effect, with length but some definition, and a navy black sheen. After consultation, we opted for a heavily cut-into shape with a hard solid fringe, and we decided to pre-lift a segment shape through the fringe before colouring the rest of the head.

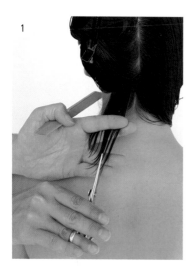

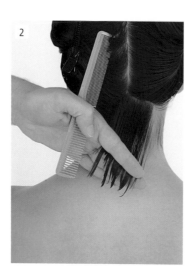

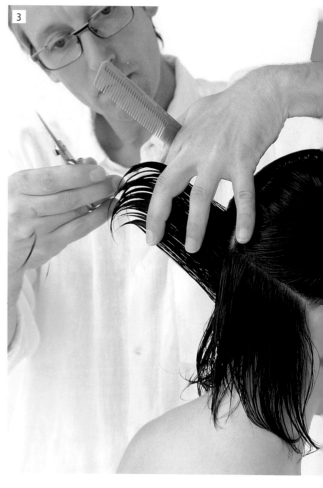

Start at the back and keep the length but cut into each section to a depth of 5–6 cm using the V-shape technique. Each section must be controlled to maintain a balance through the shape.

Continue with the technique through the back of the head up to the crown.

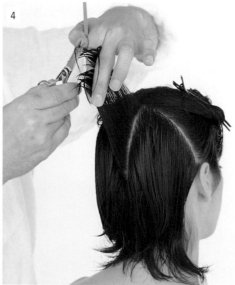

4

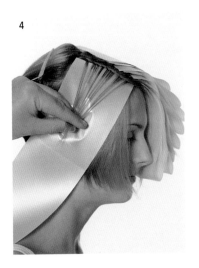

Alternate your sections between chunks of your lightest colour and slices of your other colours, with the last section being a mid-tone.

5

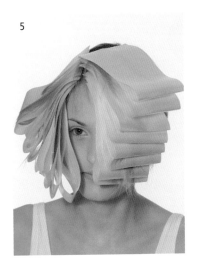

Moving to the other side, take a section parallel to the parting and set back 3 cm from the parting. Using a chunky weave, apply your lightest colour.

6

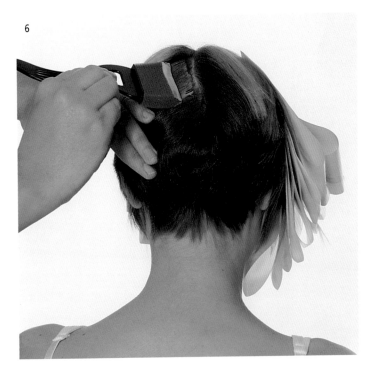

Apply a tone on tone colour to the rest of the hair, including the hair between the packets of colour. Process for 25 minutes.

Finishing

1

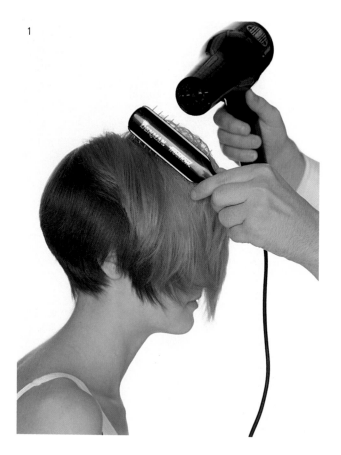

Blow-dry using a Denman vent brush, to give a smooth polished look.

2

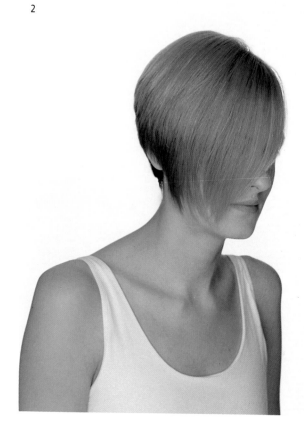

Notice how the disconnected hair through the sides and top appears visually to be checked in, but technically is not. The object of this haircut is to have a shattered outline, with no heavy weight lines. It can be worn pushed to any side, tucked behind the ears... In fact, it's a very versatile haircut!

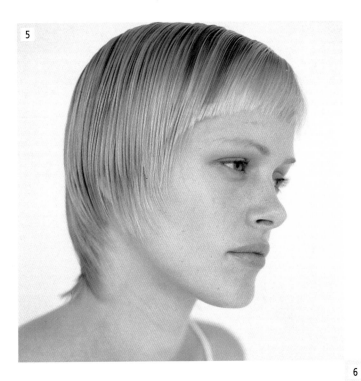

5

Side finished.

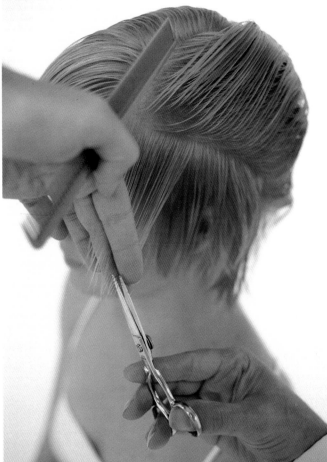

6

Cut the opposite side
in the same way.

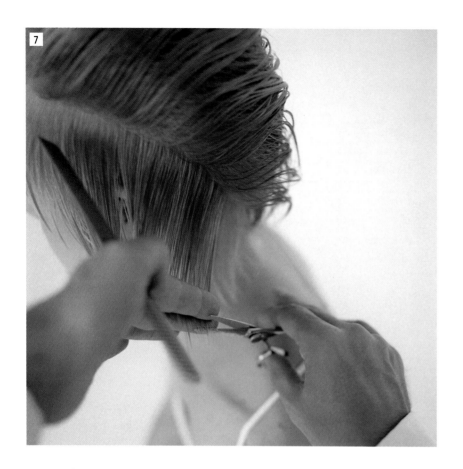

Continue line into the nape.

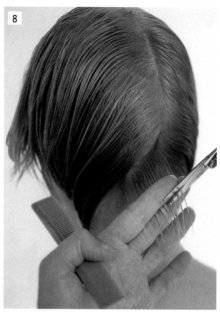

Taking horizontal sections and lifting at 45 degrees, cut a concave line into the nape hair. This creates flatness through the centre and leaves weight behind the ear.

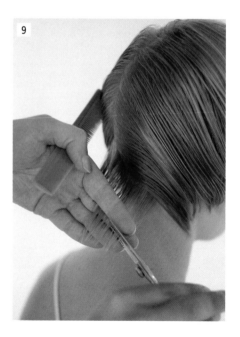

Continue this line up to 1 cm above the occipital bone.

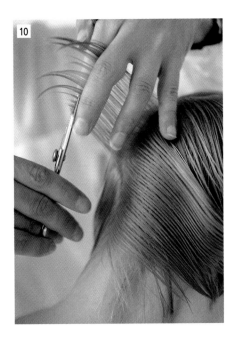

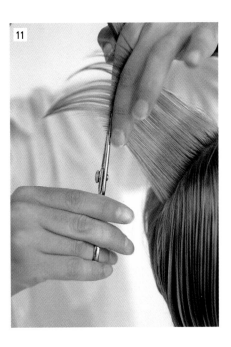

Section a panel across the back of the head, then, taking vertical sections, continue the line, keeping all your sections parallel to the head.

Section another panel across the crown and continue the line.

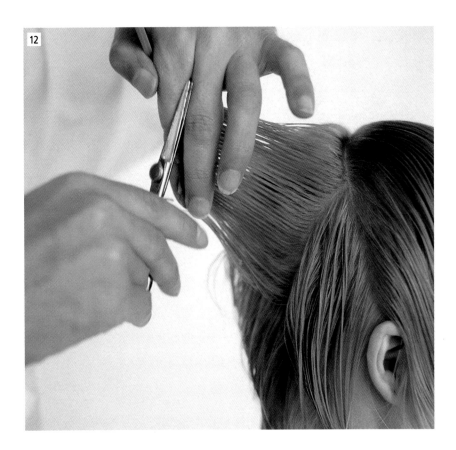

The last section is directed back to produce a square line across the back.

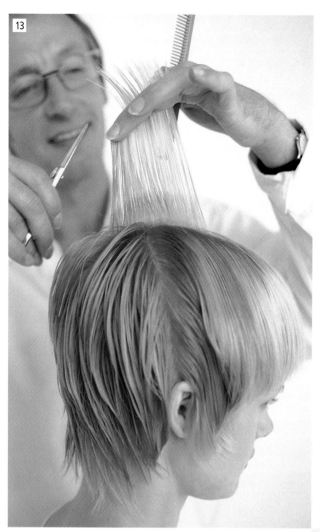

Continue your line into the top of the hair. This angle will leave length through to top front.

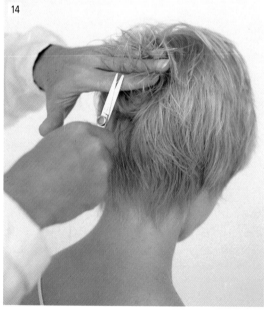

Slide your fingers across the scalp and twist through 90 degrees. This action twists the section. Slice into the remaining hair with your scissors.

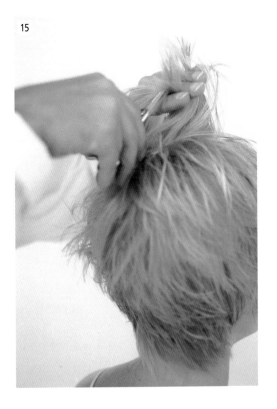

Continue this technique over the entire head.

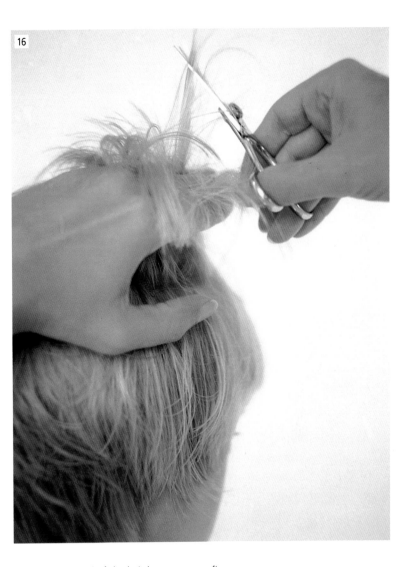

Slice away a third of the hair between your fingers.

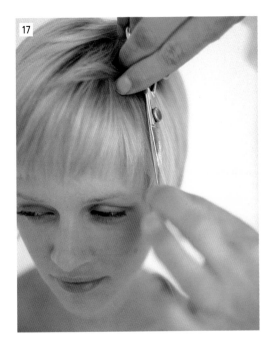

Overlay cut the fringe to produce a distressed texture. The cut is now finished.

TIPS

● The Crush will suit most face shapes as the outline layering and graduation can be customised to suit the individual.

● Overlay cutting skims off the top layer without removing the outside edge.

Colouring

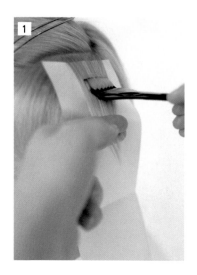

Having made two diagonal partings to form a triangle from the natural crown to the hairline, take your first section to be coloured.

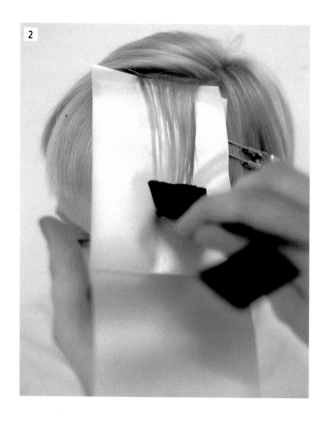

On the right side, take a slice 6 cm below the parting, approximately 4 cm wide and 1 cm deep, and apply colour using a Colour Wrap.

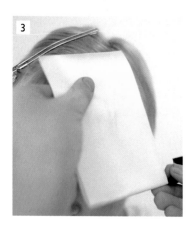

Take a slice 2 cm above the last section and repeat procedure. Then take a slice 6 cm wide at a new parting and apply colour to the section.

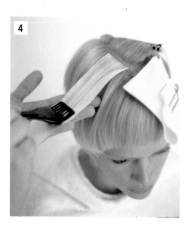

Move to the left-hand side 4 cm below the parting. Take a 6 cm slice and apply the colour. Repeat the process in another slice at the parting but reducing the width of this slice to 3 cm.

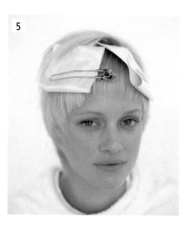

Leave to process for 20 minutes under heat/Climazon, then shampoo.

4 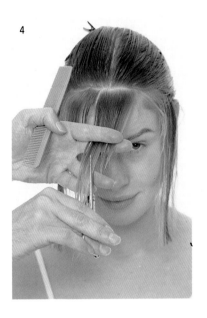 **5** 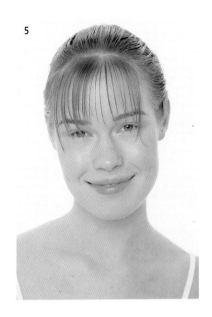 **6**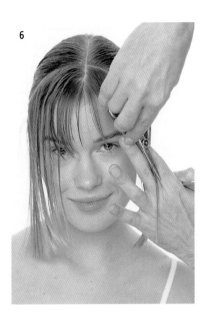

To create a long tapered fringe, cut long V-sections into the ends. Then continue a line into the side sections.

7 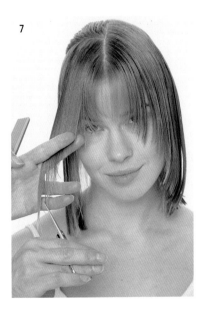 **8**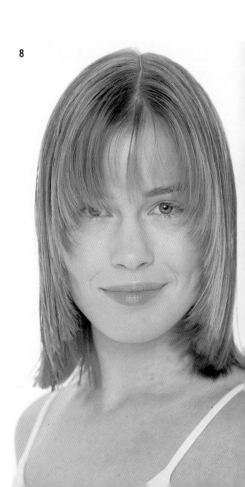

Continue your line to meet the corner, level with the front of the ear. Repeat on the opposite side.

Colouring

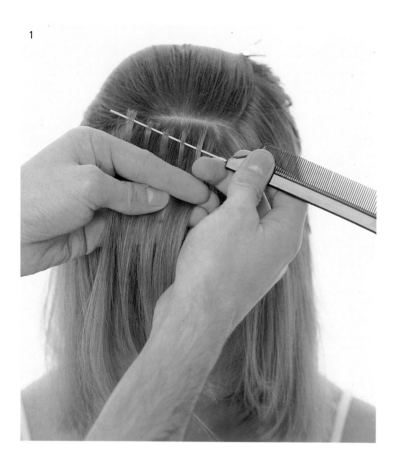

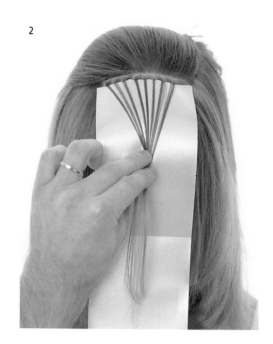

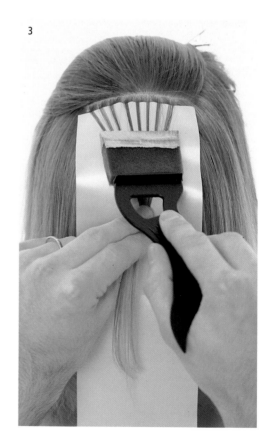

Weave out classic highlights and place them on top of the Colour Wrap.
Apply the colour with a Colour Stroker. Work through all your front sections
with this technique.

COLOUR STROKER

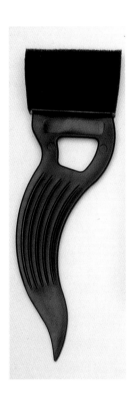

An ingenious alternative to the outdated standard tinting brush. This multifaceted hair colouring tool can be used with any hair colouring products. It has a unique ergonomic handle, and the detachable foam tips, which come in two different sizes, are soft and sensitive to the client's head. The Stroker is a quick and very efficient tool when applying tint, bleach or colour conditioner.

The Stroker can also be handy when applying hair conditioning treatments.

Why Colour Stroker?

1 Ergonomic design makes it easy and comfortable to hold and use.

2 The foam tip allows colour to be absorbed and act as a colour wall, eliminating the need to load a brush.

3 Dual action handle specially designed for easy sectioning.

4 Pack comes with four interchangeable tips of two different sizes for specific jobs.

5 Spare packs of four tips available.

6 Can be used for highlighting, partial application or full-head technique.

7 Foam tips are unaffected by colour chemicals.

8 Quick, easy application of colour due to the unique stroking action.

9 Colour is easily rinsed from the pad once the handle has been removed.

10 Feels gentle and comfortable on the scalp.

BRUSHES

The classic brush

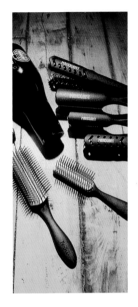

The Mahogany range of classic brushes are specially made by the highly recommended company Denman. They are available in three sizes: handbag, medium and large. They have smooth round-ended nylon pins set into a natural rubber cushion. The close-set pin formation provides exceptional grip and control, making these brushes ideal for smoothing, shaping and polishing hair.

The vent brush

The Mahogany vent brush is specially designed by Denman. This revolutionary brush incorporates a wide-spaced pin formation separated by a series of chevron vents and has a hollow brush head. This design increases the air flow to the hair, providing movement and root lift for softer, fuller hair. It is available in two sizes.

THE HAIRDRYER

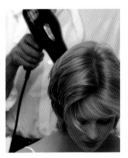

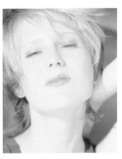

The Mahogany hairdryer is specially designed by Denman to give just the right amount of power and the right number of nozzle sizes for controlled directional drying. This British-made dryer is built of the finest materials and components. It comes with a fitted plug and a detachable concentrator and is fully guaranteed for twelve months.

WELLA PRODUCTS

HAIR COLOUR

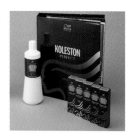

Koleston Perfect

The world's best-selling permanent hair colour. With 84 shades, Koleston Perfect has a unique synergy system to guarantee high-performance, long-lasting colour results with incredible shine.

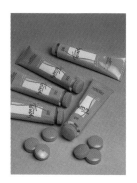

Color Touch

A long-lasting, oxidative semi-permanent colour in 34 shades with new Shine Intensive Complex – award-winning Liquid Hair and Natural Beeswax – to strengthen and condition the hair. Ideal as an introduction to colour for colour-shy clients, or for covering those initial signs of grey.

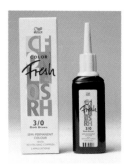

Color Fresh

A new liquid semi-permanent colour with 15 gorgeous shades which last up to 8 washes. Containing a special Revitalising Complex to condition the hair, Color Fresh is perfect as an in-between colour refresher, leaving the hair shining with health.

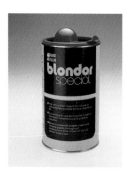

Blondor Special

A high lift, blue powder bleach for natural or coloured hair. Perfect for partial or full-head colouring techniques.

SYSTEM PROFESSIONAL

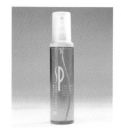

3.R Liquid Hair

Containing hydrolysed keratin – the protein found in real hair – this product works from within to restructure and strengthen, leaving the hair stronger and with more volume.

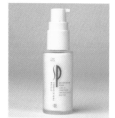

3.E Active Repair Fluid

A leave-in conditioner for the lengths and ends of the hair. It contains innovative components which form a thin, protective film around damaged ends of the hair, giving lasting protection from advanced splitting.

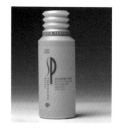

4.V Designing Fluid

A strong hold lotion for sculpting and setting. With special moisture factors to give shine and flexibility and UV filters to protect against the harmful effects of the sun.

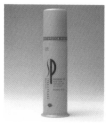

4.Y Defining Gel

A versatile gel for styling and finishing, it gives the hair superb long-lasting shine with a natural hold.

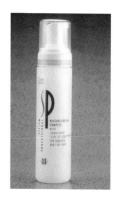

3.S Restructuring Complex with Liquid Hair

A leave-in mousse conditioner with natural hold to revitalise, condition and protect damaged or fine hair.